Iodine

Why You Need It
Why You Can't Live Without It
2ⁿᵈ Edition

For further copies of **Iodine: Why You Need It, Why You Can't Live Without It 2ⁿᵈ Edition**

Call: **1-888-647-5616** or send a check or money order in the amount of: $19.00 ($15.00 plus $4.00 shipping and handling) or for Michigan residents $19.90 ($15.00 plus $4.00 shipping and handling, plus $.90 sales tax) to:

> Medical Alternatives Press
> 4173 Fieldbrook
> West Bloomfield, Michigan 48323

Acknowledgements

I gratefully acknowledge the help I have received from my friends and colleagues in putting this book together. This book could not have been published without help from the editors—my wife Allison, Dr. Guy Abraham, Janet Darnell Dr. Rob Radtke and Tracy Hartlieb. Special thanks to Susan Bloom for all of your creative talents to design the cover. To Hailey Brownstein, thank you for all your hard work creating the title pages!

I would also like to thank my patients. It is your search for safe and effective natural treatments that is the driving force behind holistic medicine. You have accompanied me down this path and I appreciate each and every one of you.

And, to my staff. Thank you so very much for taking this trip with me. Without your help and support, none of this would be possible. I do appreciate all of your hard work and your dedication.

A Word of Caution to the Reader

The information presented in this book is based on the training and professional experience of the author. The treatments recommended in this book should not be undertaken without first consulting a physician. Proper laboratory and clinical monitoring is essential to achieving the goals of finding safe and natural treatments. This book was written for informational and educational purposes only. It is not intended to be used as medical advice.

ABOUT THE AUTHOR

David Brownstein, M.D. is a family physician who utilizes the best of conventional and alternative therapies. He is the Medical Director for the Center for Holistic Medicine in West Bloomfield, MI. He is a graduate of the University of Michigan and Wayne State University School of Medicine. Dr. Brownstein is a member of the American Academy of Family Physicians and the American College for the Advancement in Medicine. He is the father of two beautiful girls, Hailey and Jessica and is a retired soccer coach. Dr. Brownstein has lectured internationally about his success using natural items. Dr. Brownstein has authored *The Miracle of Natural Hormones 3rd Edition, Overcoming Thyroid Disorders, Overcoming Arthritis,* and *Salt Your Way to Health.*

Dr. Brownstein's office is located at:

Center for Holistic Medicine
5821 W. Maple Rd.
Ste. 192
West Bloomfield, MI 48323
248.851.1600
www.drbrownstein.com

DEDICATION

To the women of my life: Allison, Hailey and Jessica, with all my love

To physicians not satisfied with the dogma and who are willing to search for a new paradigm that promotes health.

To my staff: Thanks so much for all of your help and encouragement. I appreciate all of your hard work.

And, to my patients. Thank you for being interested in what I am interested in.

Contents

From 11th Edition of Encyclopedia Britannica 1910-1911

In medicine, iodine is frequently applied externally…and in the treatment of many conditions usually classified as surgical. The usual doses of these iodine salts are from 300mg to 900mg. Their pharmacological action is obscure just as their effects in certain diseased condition are consistently brilliant and unexampled. Our ignorance of their mode of action is cloaked by the term *deobstruent,* which implies that they possess the power of driving out impurities from the blood and tissues. The following is a list of the principal condition in which iodides are recognized to be of definite value: metallic poisonings, as by lead and mercury, asthma, aneurism, arteriosclerosis, angina pectoris, gout, goiter, syphilis, haemophillia, Bright's disease (nephritis) and bronchitis.

PREFACE

Of all the elements known so far to be essential for human health, iodine is the most misunderstood and the most feared. Yet iodine is the safest of all the essential trace elements, being the only one that can be administered safely for long periods of time to large numbers of patients in daily amounts as high as 100,000 times the RDA. However, this safety record only applies to inorganic nonradioactive forms of iodine. The reduced form of iodine is iodide with an extra electron. Based on a review of the literature, both forms, iodine/iodide are needed for optimal function of every organ and cell of the human body[1].

Some organic iodine containing drugs are extremely toxic and prescribed by physicians. The severe side effects of these drugs are blamed on inorganic iodine although studies have clearly demonstrated that it is the whole molecule that is toxic, not the iodine released from it. A case in point: the thyroid hormones are organic iodine-containing substances. Not a single physician has attributed the effects of thyroid hormones to inorganic iodine. Why not? They are basically the same forms of iodine covalently bound to an organic molecule. This author believes that this inconsistency of doublethink is most likely due to decreased cognition caused by iodine deficiency. Medical iodophobia may have caused more human misery and death than both world wars combined by preventing meaningful clinical research in the daily amount of iodine needed for optimal physical and mental health[2].

It is of interest that the recommended daily amount of iodine for supplementation by clinicians of previous generations, that is 12.5-37.5 mg in the form of Lugol's solution, turns out to be the exact range of intake for sufficiency of the whole human body, based on a recently

9

developed loading test.[3] Iodine/iodide in the proper amounts resulted in increased urinary excretion of heavy metals such as lead and mercury; and had a detoxifying effect by increasing excretion of the toxic halides fluoride and bromide.[4] It is time to wake up and realize that we are sitting on the shoulders of the giants of past generations who have given us useful information, which we have discarded in favor of preconceived ideas by self-appointed experts.

This book by Dr. David Brownstein is a welcome departure from the past and a fresh look at facts only, discarding myths and unfounded concerns about inorganic nonradioactive iodine/iodide. Patients will be grateful to Dr. Brownstein for bringing to light a simple, safe, inexpensive way of healing many medical conditions.

The ultimate Healer is the Creator of heaven and earth. His guidance has been felt constantly during this project by this author. May He bless and guide Dr. Brownstein and his patients.

"I the LORD am your healer."

(Exodus15:26)

Guy E. Abraham, M.D., FACN.

[1] Abraham, G.E., Flechas, J.D., Hakala, J.C., Orthoiodosupplementation: Iodine sufficiency of the whole human body. The Original Internist, 9:30-41, 2002.
[2] Abraham, G.E., The Wolff-Chaikoff Effect of Increasing Iodide Intake on the Thyroid. Townsend Letter, 245:100-101, 2003.
[3] Abraham, G.E. The safe and effective implementation or orthoiodosupplementation in medical practice. The Original Internist, April 2004 (In press).
[4] Abraham, G.E., Iodine Supplementation Markedly Increases Urinary Excretion of Fluoride and Bromide. Townsend Letter, 238:108-109, 2003.

Preface to the Second Edition

Less than two years ago, Dr. David Brownstein, M.D. introduced to the medical community and to consumers, his book on the essential element iodine, describing his experience with the orthoiodosupplementation program and the iodine/iodide loading test (1): simple, straightforward, and practical.

Since then, he has crisscrossed the Continental U.S.A. from East to West and North to South, lecturing on his experience with inorganic non-radioactive iodine to physicians, other healthcare professionals and consumers. Due mainly to his persistent efforts, reassuring health care professionals that inorganic non-radioactive iodine is safe and effective, there are now thousands of physicians and other health care professionals using the iodine/iodide loading test and implementing orthoiodosupplementation safely and successfully in their practices. After trying orthoiodosupplementation on themselves and their loved ones, they became confident that medical iodophobia was not justified for the inorganic, non-radioactive forms of this essential nutrient.

The number of publications presenting new research data on the orthoiodosupplementation program has increased markedly in this short time. As of December 2005, 14 manuscripts have been published (2-15). Dr. Brownstein and I coauthored a publication, reporting the positive effect of Vitamin C at 3000 mg/day on a defective cellular transport system for iodine (8), emphasizing the importance of a complete nutritional program for best results with orthoiodosupplementation. In collaboration with Drs. Brownstein and Flechas, I recently published a procedure for assessing the saliva/serum ratio of inorganic iodide as an index of the efficiency of the iodine/iodide symporter system (14). We have established normal values for the saliva/serum iodide ratio and demonstrated a negative effect of elevated serum bromide on this ratio, suggesting that bromide interferes with cellular uptake of iodide. Iodine alone in daily amounts from 50 to 100 mg iodine in the form of a Lugol tablet (Iodoral®) and Vitamin C alone at 3 gm/day both had a positive effect on the saliva/serum iodide ratio.

For the first time, a simple loading test became available to assess whole body sufficiency for iodine, the iodine/iodide loading test (5). For the first time, a simple test became available to asses the efficiency of cellular iodide uptake system using the saliva/serum stable iodide ratio (14). For the first time, the detoxifying effect of iodine at 50 mg/day on the toxic halides fluoride and bromide was reported (10). For the first time, evidence for an enterohepatic circulation of inorganic iodine was presented (11). For the first time, a mechanism used by the human body to prevent iodine overload was reported (5,7): In cases of whole body deficiency, the ingested iodine/iodide is retained by the body in proportion to the degree of deficiency. At sufficiency, the amount of iodine absorbed is quantitatively excreted in the urine as iodide, therefore protecting the body against iodine overload. In the adult, 1500 mg of iodine was retained at sufficiency (11), an amount 50 times higher than the amount of total body iodine reported in medical textbooks. We have confirmed (7) the observation of our medical predecessors (16) that iodine detoxifies the body from the heavy metals, lead and mercury (16).

The Iodine Project is now 6 years old and strong but not without enemies. Continued research and publications, education of physicians and consumers and more widespread utilization of the orthoiodosupplementation program are the most effective ways to fight iodophobic bioterrorism and medical iodophobia.

May the LORD who has faithfully guided us from the inception of this project continue to do so and bring to a close the dark age of almost 60 years which started with the Wolff-Chaikoff Effect (16,17) and which kept the importance of the essential nutrient iodine in the dark and hidden from the medical profession, causing millions to suffer and die from preventable degenerative diseases of the Western World.

Guy E. Abraham, M.D.

References

1) Brownstein, D., Iodine: *Why You Need It, Why You Can't Live Without It.* Medical Alternative Press, West Bloomfield, MI, 2004. (1-888-647-5616).
2) Abraham, G.E., Flechas, J.D., Hakala, J.C., *Optimum Levels of Iodine for Greatest Mental and Physical Health.* The Original Internist, 9:5-20, 2002.

3) Abraham, G.E., Flechas, J.D., Hakala, J.C., *Measurement of urinary iodide levels by ion-selective electrode: Improved sensitivity and specificity by chromatography on anion-exchange resin.* The Original Internist, 11(4):19-32, 2004.

4) Abraham, G.E., Flechas, J.D., Hakala, J.C., *Orthoiodosupplementation: Iodine sufficiency of the whole human body.* The Original Internist, 9:30-41, 2002.

5) Abraham, G.E., *The safe and effective implementation of orthoiodosupplementation in medical practice.* The Original Internist, 11:17-36, 2004.

6) Abraham, G.E., *The concept of orthoiodosupplementation and its clinical implications.* The Original Internist, 11(2):29-38, 2004.

7) Abraham, G.E., *The historical background of the iodine project.* The Original Internist, 12(2):57-66, 2005.

8) Abraham, G.E., Brownstein, D., *Evidence that the administration of Vitamin C improves a defective cellular transport mechanism for iodine: A case report.* The Original Internist, 12(3):125-130, 2005.

9) Abraham, G.E., *The Wolff-Chaikoff Effect: Crying Wolf?* The Original Internist, 12(3):112-118, 2005.

10) Abraham, G.E., *Iodine Supplementation Markedly Increases Urinary Excretion of Fluoride and Bromide.* Townsend Letter, 238:108-109, 2003.

11) Abraham, G.E., *Serum inorganic iodide levels following ingestion of a tablet form of Lugol solution: Evidence for an enterohepatic circulation of iodine.* The Original Internist, 11(3):29-34, 2004.

12) Brownstein, D., *Clinical experience with inorganic, non-radioactive iodine/iodide.* The Original Internist, 12(3):105-108, 2005.

13) Flechas, J.D., *Orthoiodosupplementation in a primary care practice.* The Original Internist, 12(2):89-96, 2005.

14) Abraham, G.E., Brownstein, D., Flechas, J.D., *The saliva/serum iodide ratio as an index of sodium/iodide symporter efficiency.* The Original Internist, 12(4): 152-156 , 2005.

15) Abraham, G.E., Brownstein, D., *Validation of the orthoiodosupplementation program: A Rebuttal of Dr. Gaby's Editorial on iodine.* The Original Internist, 12(4): 184-194 , 2005.

16) Encyclopedia Britannica, Vol. 11, 1910-1911-Under "Iodine".

17) Wolff, J., Chaikoff, I.L., *Plasma Inorganic Iodide as a Homeostatic Regulator of Thyroid Function.* J. Biol. Chem., 174:555-564, 1948.

18) Wolff, J., *Iodide Goiter and the Pharmacologic Effects of Excess Iodide.* Am. J. Med., 47:101-124, 1969.

FOREWORD

Practicing holistic medicine for over 10 years has brought me into contact with many wonderful teachers. From these people I have learned a tremendous amount about how to use safe and natural remedies to promote true healing in the body while not relying on foreign substances (i.e., drugs) that simply treat the symptoms of illness and do little for treatment of the underlying cause of illness.

There are many physicians that I have learned from. Some of these wonderful physicians who have researched and educated others about their successes in using natural items to promote true healing include Jonathan Wright, Majid Ali, Broda Barnes and William Jeffries. There are many more.

I would like to add one more name to that list. His name is Guy Abraham. Dr. Abraham has been researching the benefits of iodine therapy for 6 years. Dr. Abraham began studying the effects of iodine and looking at the research on iodine therapy. He has written numerous articles about the misinformation on iodine and how this misinformation has contributed to the poor health of many of us.

While reading ***The Townsend Letter for Doctors and Patients (May, 2003)***, I read a letter to the editor that was titled, "Iodine Supplementation Markedly Increases Urinary Excretion of Fluoride and Bromide". I was intrigued. I knew of the deficiency of iodine and the consequences of this deficiency. I was also aware of certain toxic items (i.e., fluoride and bromide) in our diet that not only inhibited iodine utilization in the body but also accentuated an iodine deficiency. After reading Dr. Abraham's letter, I phoned him.

I expressed my interest in iodine testing and treatment and Dr. Abraham began to educate me about how to test for iodine and how to properly use iodine. Since that time, I have tested hundreds of patients and found a significant number (>90%) exhibit laboratory signs of iodine deficiency. Treatment with the correct amount and correct form of iodine has greatly contributed to the good health of many of these patients.

Dr. Abraham and I have been collaborating for many months now. He is one physician (amongst many) who is not afraid to stand up and report what he thinks is true, even if it does not sit well with the establishment. But, Dr. Abraham uses good science to back up his claims. After pulling hundreds of research articles to educate myself, I realized that Dr. Abraham's view of iodine deficiency was 100% correct.

This book certainly would not have been written without the help and research of Dr. Abraham. I have learned a tremendous amount from Dr. Abraham and I can't thank him enough.

David Brownstein, M.D.
April, 2004

FOREWORD to the 2nd Edition

It has now been 18 months since the publishing of the first edition of ***Iodine: Why You Need It, Why You Can't Live Without It.*** Since then, a great deal of new information has come forward, all building on the basic premises of the first book.

At my office, we (Drs. Brownstein, Nusbaum and Ng) have now tested and treated over 3,000 patients with iodine. The results still amaze me. Iodine deficiency is rampant. Over 95% of those tested have demonstrated low iodine levels.

With iodine supplementation, hypothyroid and autoimmune thyroid symptoms improve. Cancer therapies are more effective when iodine deficiency is rectified.   Autoimmune disorders clinically improve with iodine supplementation. Most importantly, people feel better when the body is given the proper form and amounts of iodine.

The reason there is so much iodine deficiency present is not only due to inadequate iodine intake, it is also due to the toxicities we are exposed to on a daily basis. These toxicities include the toxic halides bromine, fluoride and the chlorine derivatives. This book will provide more information about how these halides are adversely affecting not only our body's iodine status but our immune system as well.

It still astounds me how much misinformation there is about iodine. This occurs with physicians and lay people alike. The "wives tale" that we get enough iodine in iodized salt has been parroted for over 50 years. This "wives tale" is false. The research is clear; iodized salt is a poor source of iodide as it is not bioavailable for the body (see Chapter 2).

Iodine deficiency is widespread. Conventional medicine has failed to understand this fact. However, with increased research, the truth will come out. It has to. There is no alternative physiology or alternative biochemistry. Science does not lie. Iodine deficiency does occur in today's world and it is occurring at very high levels.

Correcting iodine deficiency has proven to have many positive health benefits. Ensuring adequate iodine levels helps prevent and treat autoimmune illnesses, thyroid disorders, cancer and other conditions. This book will educate the reader on the benefits of the remarkable nutrient iodine.

TO ALL OF OUR HEALTH,

David Brownstein
January, 2006

Chapter 1

Introduction to Iodine

CHAPTER 1: INTRODUCTION TO IODINE

Steven, a 55-year-old photographer, complained of losing his creative abilities. "I can't see the pictures like I used to. In fact, I have no motivation to even work. I feel like I am in a fog," he claimed. Steven was diagnosed with depression three years earlier and treated with antidepressant medications. Although he felt some improvement from the antidepressant medications, he found that he was having difficulty being productive at work. "My business was going down the tubes. Clients were leaving me left and right," he claimed. When I saw Steven, he had many of the signs of hypothyroidism including poor eyebrow growth, slow reflexes, puffiness under his eyes, and very dry skin. Steven's blood tests showed low-normal thyroid function tests and a very low basal body temperature (96.6 degrees Fahrenheit—normal 97.8-98.2 degrees Fahrenheit). Steven's iodine-loading test showed a low iodine level at 23% excretion (normal: >90% excretion. The iodine-loading test will be explained in Chapter 2). He was initially treated with 50mg/day of iodine/iodide (Iodoral®). His blood and hair tests revealed nutritional deficiencies that were contributing to his problems. He was treated with a combination of vitamins, minerals, and unrefined salt (Celtic Sea Salt®), in addition to the iodine. At a two-month follow-up visit, he reported, "I am so much better. It is like night and day. My creative level is tremendously improved. I can now see things at work. You either have the eye for photography or you don't. Now I have it again. I feel like I am 20 years old. Now, my phone won't stop ringing. The only bad thing is that I am getting too busy."

Steven's story is not unique. The human body is a wonderful thing. If you give it the proper nutrients, it can perform optimally. Conversely, when the raw materials (vitamins, minerals, hormones, enzymes, amino acids, etc.) are lacking or imbalanced, it sets the stage for poor health and the onset of disease. At the present time, iodine deficiency is occurring at epidemic proportions. This book will explore the causes and treatment of iodine deficiency.

WHAT DOES IODINE DO?

For over 100 years, iodine has been known as the element that is necessary for thyroid hormone production. However, it is rare to see any further mention of iodine's other effects in the body. Iodine is found in each of the trillions of cells in the body. Without adequate iodine levels, life itself is not possible.

Iodine is not only necessary for the production of thyroid hormone, it is also responsible for the production of all of the other hormones of the body. Adequate iodine levels are necessary for proper immune system function. Iodine contains potent antibacterial, antiparasitic, antiviral, and anticancer properties. Iodine is also effective for treating fibrocystic breasts and ovarian cysts. Table 1 lists some of the many benefits of iodine and some of the conditions that would benefit from adequate iodine supplementation. This book will review the many therapeutic aspects of iodine.

Approximately 1.5 billion people, about one-third of the earth's population, live in an area of iodine deficiency as defined by the World Health Organization. Iodine deficiency disorder can result in mental retardation, goiter, increased child and infant mortality, infertility, and socioeconomic decline.[1] Iodine deficiency disorder is the most common preventable form of mental retardation known.

Table 1: Therapeutic Actions of Iodine and Conditions Iodine Can Treat

Therapeutic Actions	Conditions Treated With Iodine
Antibacterial	ADD
Anticancer	Breast Diseases
Antiparasitic	Dupuytren's Contracture
Antiviral	Excess Mucous Production
Mucolytic Agent	Fatigue
	Fibrocystic Breasts
	Hemorrhoids
	Headaches
	Keloids
	Migraine Headaches
	Ovarian Disease
	Parotid Duct Stones
	Peyronie's
	Sebaceous Cysts
	Thyroid Disorders
	Vaginal Infections

Iodine is a relatively rare element, ranking 62nd in abundance of the elements of the earth. Iodine is primarily found in seawater in very small quantities and solid rocks (usually near the ocean) that form when seawater evaporates. Iodine can also be found in sea organisms, such as seaweed. In fact, seaweed is one of the most abundant sources of iodine because seaweed has the ability to concentrate a large amount of iodine from the ocean water.

Iodine is not very abundant in the earth's crust. It is estimated to be about 0.3-0.5 parts per million. In fact, it is in the bottom third of the elements in terms of abundance.[2]

If the soil has adequate iodine levels, the crops grown on that soil will contain adequate iodine levels. Conversely, deficient iodine levels will be found in crops grown on iodine-deficient soil.

There are naturally occurring non-radioactive and radioactive forms of iodine. Radioactive iodine can be used in medicine to diagnose and treat certain illnesses, particularly illnesses of the thyroid gland.

Commercially available non-radioactive iodine primarily comes from several sources: Chilean Saltpeter, seaweed, and brine water in oil wells. The action of the waves from the ocean can make iodine gas. Once airborne, iodine can combine with water or air and enter the soil. Non-radioactive iodine can enter our food system in a variety of ways. First, plants can take up iodine from the soil. Second, airborne iodine can land on fresh water supplies and, finally, airborne iodine can land on the ground, combine with salt, and become iodized salt.

Radioactive iodine can enter the air from reactions in nuclear power plants or explosions of nuclear materials. Radioactive iodine has been associated with certain types of cancer including thyroid cancer and certain blood cancers. Children are more susceptible to radioactive iodine since they have smaller thyroid glands, and they will receive a proportionately larger radioactive dose than an adult when they are exposed to radioactive iodine. Radioactive iodine damage can be prevented by the ingestion of non-radioactive inorganic iodine.

WHERE IS IODINE FOUND IN THE BODY?

Every cell in the body contains and utilizes iodine. Iodine is concentrated in the glandular system of the body. The thyroid gland contains a higher concentration of iodine than any other organ of the body. Large amounts of iodine are also stored in many other areas of the body including the salivary glands, cerebrospinal fluid and the brain[3], gastric mucosa, choroid plexus, breasts, ovaries, and the ciliary body of the eye. In the brain, iodine concentrates in the substantia nigra, an area of the brain that has been associated with Parkinson's disease.

Iodine is essential for the normal growth and development of children. Severe iodine deficiency can result in severe mental deficiency and deafness (i.e., cretinism). In addition, spontaneous abortion, as well as delayed physical and intellectual development is associated with iodine deficiency.

Conversely, too much iodine can be a problem. In rare cases, excess iodine (i.e., doses greater than 1gram/day) has been associated with hyperthyroid symptoms.

28

HISTORY OF IODINE

Bernard Courtois first discovered iodine in 1811 during the course of making gunpowder.[4] He was making compounds of potassium and sodium from seaweed. When he accidentally added too much sulphuric acid to the mixture, he observed purple vapors arising from it. Due to its purple color, the new element was named iodine (iodes in Greek means violet). [5]

The first medical use of iodine was reported by Jean Francois Coindet (1774-1834), who showed that goiter (i.e., swelling of the thyroid) could be treated with iodine. The use of iodine in treating goiter was the first time that a single item (iodine) was used to treat a specific illness (goiter). Some cite this discovery as the birth of western medicine.

Jean-Baptiste Boussingault (1802-1887) verified the work of Coindet in 1824. Boussingault observed that goiter did not occur at many silver mining sites. His experiments showed conclusively that iodine in the water at these mining sites prevented goiter in people who drank the water. His recommendation at the time was that goiter could be prevented by having people eat the iodine-containing salt from these mines.

MICHIGAN/OHIO STUDIES

In the early 1900's there was a high prevalence of goiter in the states bordering the Great Lakes. Due to the earlier work of Boussingault and Coindet, it was hypothesized that adding iodine to the diet of people in the Great Lakes area would decrease the incidence of goiter. In 1923-1924, the State of Michigan's Department of Health conducted a large-scale survey of goiter in four counties. Of 66,000 school children examined, nearly 40% had enlargement of the thyroid gland (i.e., goiter).[6][7][8] In 1924, iodized salt was introduced to the area. By 1928, there was a 75% reduction of goiter observed and by 1951, less than 0.5% of school-age children had a goiter. Research also showed a greater reduction in goiter among regular users of iodized salt as compared to non-users.

David Marine conducted the first large-scale study on using iodine as a therapy to reduce goiter. In the early 1900's, he looked at the positive effects of iodine supplementation decreasing goiter in farm animals. He estimated the amount of iodine necessary to treat humans.

Dr. Marine chose Akron, Ohio as the test area for iodine supplementation. Akron, Ohio was chosen due to the high rate of goiter—56% of school-aged girls had goiter in Akron.[9] There was a 600% increase in goiter in adolescent girls versus boys.[10] Dr. Marine studied two groups of students:

1. A control group of 2305 students where no iodine was given.

2. A treatment group of 2190 students who were given 9mg/day of sodium iodide (averaged daily) for 2.5 years. This dose of iodine is nearly 100x the present RDA for iodine.

The results are shown below. The control group (no iodine) showed a 22% incidence of goiter. The treatment group had a significantly lowered 0.2% incidence of goiter.

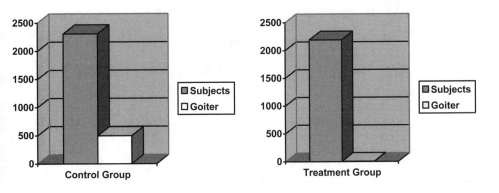

Due to the positive results from using iodized salt in Michigan and Ohio, the rest of the United States quickly adopted the policy of adding iodine to salt, thus decreasing the goiter rate throughout the country. Today, the World Health Organization actively promotes the use of iodized salt to help prevent goiter throughout the world.

HOW DO YOU INGEST IODINE?

Iodine, unlike vitamins and minerals, is not present in adequate amounts in most foods. Specific plants absorb iodine when it is present in the soil. Iodine is found in many ocean foods, such as fish (cod, sea bass, haddock, and perch) and sea vegetables (seaweed). Iodine can also be found in many other food products either by adding iodine to animal feed or by adding iodine to the food source.

Iodine has also been added to salt products (i.e., iodized salt). The U.S. government determined that the most cost-effective way to prevent goiter of the thyroid gland was to add iodine to the salt supply. Although the addition of iodine to the salt supply has lessened the prevalence of goiter, it is inadequate to supply the body's need for iodine. This will be more fully explained in Chapter 2.

HOW MUCH IODINE IS IN SALT?

Iodine is added to table salt at 100ppm as potassium iodide, which amounts to 77ug iodine/gram of salt. Estimates are that 50% of the U.S. population uses iodized table salt.[11] However, that estimate is probably high due to the prevalence of low-salt diets and low-salt food products. Chapter 2 will explore this topic in more detail.

The amount of iodine in food varies. Seafood, multiple vitamins, and many farm products may contain iodine. Dairy products, eggs, and meat may contain iodine if iodine is properly added to the feed of animals. Table 2 lists the iodine content of many different food sources. However, iodine was removed from many food products in the 1980's and these estimates may not be valid today.

Table 2: Iodine Content in Some Food Items in the United States (1982-1989)

Food	µg/iodine/serving
Ready to eat cereals	87
Dairy-based desserts	70
Fish	57
Milk	56
Overall dairy products	49
Eggs	27
Bread	27
Beans, peas, tuber	17
Meat	16
Poultry	15

1990 Iron, zinc, copper, manganese, selenium and iodine in foods from the United States total diet study. J. Food Compos. Anal. 3:166

WHY THE SOIL IS DEFICIENT IN IODINE

The soil around the oceans generally contains adequate amounts of iodine. The more inland and mountainous areas generally have lesser amounts of iodine. The Midwestern United States, including my home state, Michigan, is part of the "Goiter

Belt" since our soils are so deficient in iodine. The Goiter Belt is not close to any natural iodine-containing source (i.e., ocean). Any natural or man-made phenomenon that leads to soil erosion will make an iodine-deficient soil problem worse. The movement of the glaciers across the Midwest is cited as one of the reasons why the soil is iodine deficient. In addition, deforestation and poor farming techniques exacerbate this problem.

This book will explore, in detail, the medical conditions that can arise as a result of iodine deficiency and how these disorders can be improved by supplementing with the correct amount and form of iodine. The next two case histories give examples of some of the conditions that can be treated with iodine supplementation.

Kevin, a 31-year-old sales representative, was well until he had a flu shot one year ago. "Before receiving that vaccination, I was an extremely active weight lifter for 12 years. After the flu shot, I became disabled. I could not work and I could barely get out of bed in the morning," he said. Kevin was diagnosed with hypothyroidism shortly after the flu shot and put on Synthroid. When I saw Kevin, he had many of the signs of hypothyroidism, including puffiness, dry skin, thickened tongue, and slow reflexes. I changed Kevin's medication to Armour thyroid and he noticed an immediate improvement, but he still did not feel like his normal self. Laboratory tests showed that Kevin was extremely iodine deficient (24-hour loading test showed 55% iodine excretion— normal >90% excretion. The iodine-loading test is explained in

Chapter 2). After supplementing with an iodine/iodide supplement, he noticed an immediate improvement. He was feeling so much better that he wrote me a letter which said:

"In the first five weeks of taking the iodine, I lost five pounds. The weights that I have been able to use on practically all of my exercises have increased between 15-25%. My recuperation time between workouts seems to be steadily improving. It seems as though I have been waking up on time much more consistently than ever before. I am awake and energized at about 6:00 a.m., which has never been the case before in my life! Additionally, I feel as though my energy level is much more stable throughout the day. Since I have been taking the iodine, my need for caffeine in the morning has disappeared. Overall Dr. Brownstein, I feel much better than I did before starting the iodine therapy."

Paula, age 42, suffered with severe headaches for over ten years. "I almost learned to live with the headaches. They just became a daily part of my life," she said. Paula was being treated for hypothyroidism with Armour thyroid and noticed the thyroid hormone improved her headaches by approximately 40%. Paula said, "I was happy to get some relief, but I wasn't satisfied. It is no fun to wake up most days with a vice around your head." When Paula was checked for iodine levels, her serum iodine levels were zero (below the detectable limits of the test). The low iodine levels were confirmed with an iodine-loading test (explained in Chapter 2) which was extremely low at 17% (normal >90%). Paula was placed on 37.5mg of a combination of iodine and iodide

(Iodoral®) and noticed an improvement in her headaches within two weeks. "I couldn't believe it. I started to actually have headache-free days. After four weeks on the iodine, my headaches were over 95% better. When I had a headache, it wasn't nearly as severe. As I started to feel better, I began to realize how much the headaches were impacting my life," she claimed. Paula ran out of the iodine two months later and all of her symptoms began returning. Paula reported, "It took about two weeks off of the iodine before the headaches started to return. All of the same symptoms I was suffering with began to come back. Again, after I started the iodine, the headaches began to go away. I feel like the iodine has given me a new lease on life. My husband and my children thank you."

[1] Manner, M.G., et al. Salt Iodization for the Elimination of Iodine Deficiency. International Council for the Control of Iodine Deficiency Disorders. 1995

[2] Modern Nutrition in Health and Disease, 9th Edition. Williams and Wilkins, 1999.

[3] Adrasi, E. Iodine concentration in different human brain parts. Analytical and Bioanalytical chemistry. November 13, 2003

[4] Modern Nutrition in Health and Disease, 9th Edition. Williams and Wilkins, 1999.

[5] Newton, David. Chemical Elements. Lawrence W. Baker, Editor. 1999

[6] Kimball, O.P. Prevention of goiter in Michigan and Ohio. JAMA. 1937; 108:860-864

[7] Matovinovic, J., et al. Goiter and other thyroid disease in Tecumseh, Michigan. JAMA. 1965: 192(#): 134-140

[8] Kimball, O.P. Endemic Goiter: A food deficiency disease. J. Am. Dietetic. Assn. 1949; 25:112

[9] Marine, D. Prevention and treatment of simple goiter. Atl. Med. J. 26:437-442, 1923

[10] Marine, D. The prevention of simple goiter in man. J . Lab. Clin. Med. 3:40-48

[11] Dunn, John. Editorial: What's happening to our iodine? J. of Clinical Endcrin. And Metab. Vol. 83, No. 10. 1998

Chapter 2

Why are Iodine Levels so Low?

CHAPTER 2: WHY ARE IODINE LEVELS SO LOW?

David, a 42-year-old Michigander, had taken good care of himself. He regularly took vitamins and minerals, did not eat a lot of junk food and exercised regularly. "I feel better now than I did when I was in my 20's. I eat better and my energy level is better," he said. His father, mother and two sisters were being treated for hypothyroidism. David was diagnosed with hypothyroidism eight years ago and was taking thyroid medication (Armour® thyroid) regularly. When David's iodine level was checked with an iodine/iodide loading test, he was shocked. His iodine level was found to be very low at 46.2% excretion (normal excretion is greater than 90%). "I couldn't believe it. How could my iodine level be so low, when I felt so good? I have been taking vitamins and minerals for years," he said. When he started supplementing *with an iodine/iodide combination (Iodoral®), he immediately felt better. "My energy level dramatically increased. I thought I was feeling good before I began taking the iodine, but now I know what really feeling good is about. I started sleeping better and my dreams became much more vivid. In addition, my head felt much clearer. It feels wonderful," he exclaimed. After three months of iodine supplementation, David's iodine levels improved to a more healthy 87% excretion (normal levels >90%).*

David is your author. After experiencing the wonderful effects of taking iodine, and hearing of the positive results my patients have experienced with using iodine, I became very interested in researching its clinical uses.

INTRODUCTION

Iodine deficiency is a worldwide problem. Diets that are deficient in iodine can result in many severe medical conditions including cretinism (very severe brain damage occurring in very early life), mental impairment, reduced intellectual ability, goiter, and infertility. In addition, iodine deficiency predisposes one to an increased risk of breast, prostate, endometrial, and ovarian cancer.[1] There is a decreased childhood survival rate associated with iodine deficiency. Studies have shown that neonatal mortality can be decreased by up to 50% when iodine deficiency is rectified.[2] Other illnesses that may result from iodine deficiency include sudden infant death syndrome (SIDS), multiple sclerosis, and other myelin disorders.[3]

The World Health Organization has recognized that iodine deficiency is the world's greatest single cause of preventable mental retardation.[4] Iodine deficiency has been identified as a significant public health problem in 129 countries. Approximately one-third of the world's population lives in iodine deficient areas and up to 72% of the world's population is affected by an iodine deficiency disorder.[5]

IODIZED SALT

Some may think that the iodization of salt (i.e., iodized salt) has eliminated iodine deficiency disorders in the United States. However, the data does not support that conclusion. Over the last 30 years, studies by the National Health and Nutrition Examination Survey I (NHANES—completed 1971-1974) and NHANES 2000 show iodine levels have dropped 50% in the United States (see figure on next page).[6] This drop was seen in all demographic categories: ethnicity, region, economic status, population density, and race. The percentage of pregnant women with low iodine concentrations increased 690% over this time period. As previously mentioned, low iodine concentrations in pregnant women have been shown to increase the risk for cretinism, mental retardation, attention deficit disorder, and other health issues in children.

NATIONAL HEALTH AND NUTRITION EXAMINATION SURVEY IODIDE LEVELS

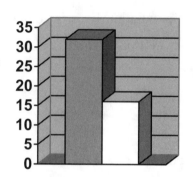

HOW MUCH IODINE IS IN IODIZED SALT?

In the United States, iodine is added to salt to provide a content of 77µg of iodine per gm of salt.[7] Although the content of iodine in salt varies from country to country (depending on the standard set by the governing agencies), the goal is to achieve the RDA for iodine. In the United States, the RDA of iodine is from 150µg/day to 290µg/day (see Table 3). The average salt intake in the U.S.A. is estimated to be approximately 10g/day, which would theoretically supply 770µg of iodine. However, studies have shown that urine levels of iodine in 24-hour urine tests are ten times lower.[8]

Table 3: RDA for Iodine[9]
The recommended daily allowance of iodine

Life Stage	RDA
Adult Male	150µg/d
Adult Female	150µg/d
Pregnancy	220µg/d
Lactation	290µg/d

Remember, the RDA for iodine was set up to prevent goiter, which it does very well. However, as illustrated in this chapter, the RDA for iodine is inadequate to fully supply the rest of the body's needs for a properly functioning thyroid gland, cancer prevention, an optimal immune system, and other vital functions for the body.

IS IODIZED SALT A GOOD SOURCE OF IODINE?

As mentioned above, iodine levels have fallen by approximately 50% over the last 30 years according to the NHANES data.[10] Iodine was added to salt in the 1920's to help combat thyroid goiter. Since that time, iodine is still being added to salt.

I was taught in medical school that there is enough iodine in salt to supply the body's need for iodine. In fact, this has been taught in every medical school for over 80 years. However, there were no studies to back up this claim and the NHANES data clearly shows that there is something happening to cause iodine levels to decrease 50% over the last 30 years.

Is salt the best source of iodine for the body? The research does not support the idea that salt is a readily available source of iodine for the body.

In 1969, researchers looked at the bioavailability of iodine in salt versus bread.[11] Two groups of people were studied; one group ingested a measured amount of iodine in salt, the other group ingested a measured amount of iodine in bread. Both subject groups were estimated to ingest approximately 750mcg of iodine. By ingesting 750mcg of iodine, the expected serum levels of iodine would be 17.2µg/L. However, as shown in the figure below, the iodized salt group only had a serum level of 1.7µg/L. versus 18.7µg/L for the bread group. This information would suggest that iodized salt is only 10% bioavailable.[12]

Bioavailabiltiy of Iodide in Salt

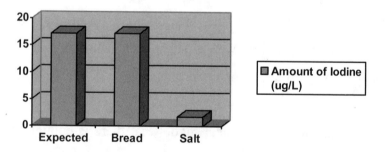

46

Iodine is added primarily to refined salt. Refined salt is a lifeless product that has had all of its minerals removed and has been exposed to toxic chemicals that gives it its white color. As I explained in my book, ***Salt Your Way to Health***, the ingestion of refined salt leads to many health problems. Unrefined salt should be the salt-of-choice. For more information on the health benefits of unrefined salt, I refer the reader to ***Salt Your Way to Health.***

WHY ARE PEOPLE DEFICIENT IN IODINE?

It has been assumed that since the iodization of salt was implemented, iodine deficiency disorders would be a thing of the past. Due to the poor availability of iodine in salt as well as a declining salt intake by the population, this is not the case. There are additional reasons why iodine deficiency disorders are still present today.

Due to poor farming techniques, deficiencies of iodine and other minerals in the soil have increased. Crops grown in iodine-deficient soil will be deficient in iodine. Also, the stigma of salt causing high blood pressure has convinced many individuals not to use salt in their foods. Many times the only iodine one will get from the diet is found in salt. A low-salt diet can naturally lead to an iodine-deficient state.

Radioactive iodine, used in many medical procedures, will further exacerbate an iodine deficiency problem. Also, exposure to many chemicals that inhibit iodine binding in the body (e.g.,

47

bromide, fluoride, chloride—explained in Chapter 5) further worsens the problem.

Certain diets and lifestyles can also predispose one to developing iodine deficiency. Some examples of these diets are listed below. Inadequate dietary iodine intake can cause many severe problems including thyroid problems, cancer, intellectual decline, cretinism, and others.

Diets That May Cause Iodine Deficiency
1. Diets without ocean fish or sea vegetables
2. Inadequate use of iodized salt including low-sodium diets
3. Diets high in the consumption of bakery products (e.g., breads, pasta) which contain bromide
4. Vegan and vegetarian diets

The most significant change in the iodine status of recent time occurred with the changing of the food industry. In the 1960's, iodine was added to the commercial baking industry as a dough conditioner. This single addition to baked goods significantly increased the iodine intake of the U.S. population, as one slice of bread contained the RDA for iodine of 150ug.[13] Articles from the NIH were published which questioned the safety of using iodine in baking products. Some researchers felt that this level of iodine in baking products would cause a malfunctioning of the thyroid gland.

Twenty years later, bromine replaced iodine in the baking industry. Bromine is a halide (as is iodine, fluoride, and chloride). All halides compete with one another for absorption and receptor binding in the body. Bromine interferes with iodine utilization in the thyroid as well as wherever else iodine would concentrate in the body.[14]

Due to the interference of iodine binding in the body, bromine is a known "goitrogen"—it promotes the formation of goiter in the body. Bromine is a toxic substance that has no therapeutic use in our bodies. Bromine also can bind to iodine receptors in the breast and is a known carcinogen to the breast. On the other hand, iodine has anticarcinogenic properties.

We now have two major reasons why iodine deficiency disorders have become much more common.

1. The substitution of bromine for iodine in the bakery process lowered the iodine utilization.
2. Bromine began effectively binding to and inhibiting iodine from binding to its own receptors.

The consequence of replacing iodine with bromine has been to make a bad situation worse. Iodine deficiency has been accelerated and iodine is now inhibited from binding to its own receptors. The medical consequences include increased thyroid disorders including autoimmune thyroid disorders (Hashimoto's and Graves' disease), and thyroid cancer. In addition, the rise of other cancers including breast and prostate cancer may be related to this phenomenon. This will be explained further in Chapters 4 and 5.

PERCHLORATE

Perchlorate is a substance that is found in nature and is a man-made substance. Perchlorate is manufactured for rocket fuel and many industrial uses. Perchlorate contains one atom of chlorine and four atoms of oxygen. Chlorine is part of the halide family (iodine, bromine and chlorine). Excess perchlorate levels can displace iodine in the body and damage the transport of iodine into the cell. Perchlorate contamination of our water supply is widespread and increasing. Increasing perchlorate exposure is another reason why iodine levels have fallen over the last 30 years. Chapter 5 reviews the details and consequences of perchlorate exposure in much more detail.

HOW DO YOU MEASURE IODINE LEVELS?

The generally accepted method of testing iodine levels is by measuring the amount of iodine in the urine. However, that is not a reliable method.

Recently, Dr. Abraham and coinvestigators have developed an iodine-loading test that is based on the concept that the more iodine deficiency there is, the more iodine is retained in the body and the less iodine is excreted in the urine.[15] The iodine-loading test has been found to provide very useful information on the body's iodine status.

Iodine binds to iodine receptors throughout the body. If the body's receptors for iodine are sufficient in iodine, a large percentage of ingested iodine will be excreted from the body. On the other hand, if there is an iodine deficiency present, ingested iodine will be retained at a much larger percentage.

The iodine-loading test is performed after taking 50mg of an iodine/iodide combination. Urine is collected for 24 hours after taking the iodine. In an iodine sufficient state, approximately 90% of a mixture of a 50mg dose of iodine/iodide would be excreted (i.e., 45mg), and 10% of the iodine would be retained (i.e., 5mg). Levels below 90% excretion would indicate an iodine-deficient state.

FIRST LOOK AT IODINE LEVELS AT MY OFFICE

Twenty-four patients in my office were selected at random to have their iodine status evaluated. Each patient was instructed to take 50mg of a combination of iodine/iodide (Iodoral®) and collect 24 hours of urine. The urine was evaluated for the amount of iodine excreted. The results (Figure 1) show that 91.7% of the patients tested low for iodine levels. Iodine sufficiency occurs when the urinary excretion is above 90%.

FIGURE 1: IODINE LEVELS IN 24 PATIENTS

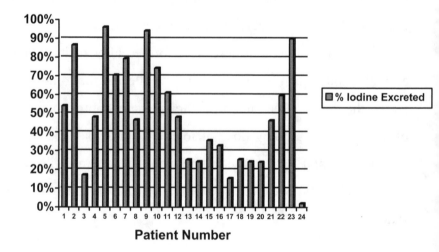

Patient Number

Most of the patients studied had thyroid abnormalities, including hypothyroidism, Hashimoto's, or Graves' disease. There was no difference in the iodine levels between the various thyroid disorders; most were low. In fact, almost all patients, regardless of their condition, were low in iodine. This study shows how widespread iodine deficiency is.

UPDATED RESULTS AT MY OFFICE

To the present date, we have now tested iodine levels in well over 1,000 patients. Our results have been consistent; over 90% of patients test low for iodine. Dr. Jorge Flechas, the owner of FFP labs (see Appendix for more information on FFP labs) has been at the forefront of testing people world-wide for their iodine levels. His results are consistent with mine. Dr. Flechas' tested over 4,000 patients and his results are shown below. They are consistent with my results. His data shows that the mean urinary iodide excretion after ingesting 50mg of iodine/iodide (Iodoral®) was 19.78μg/L (normal levels >45μg/L).

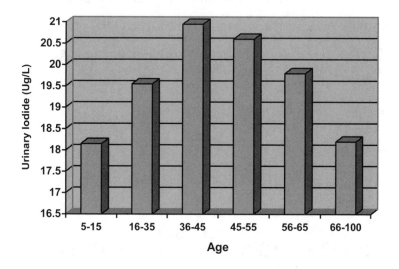

Iodide Loading Test in 4065 Patients (Mean 19.78ug/L--normal 45ug/L). From FFP Lab

FINAL THOUGHTS

Iodine deficiency is a huge public health problem. The exposure to goitrogens (substances that promote goiter), including the halides bromide and fluoride, has exacerbated the iodine deficiency problem. It is one of the main underlying causes of many varied illnesses including thyroid disorders, chronic fatigue, fibromyalgia, cancer (including cancer of the breast and prostate), and other health issues. I believe that properly evaluating and treating iodine deficiency will not only help people improve the functioning of their immune systems, but it will also be an integral part of achieving their optimal health.

[1] Stadel, B. Dietary iodine and risk of breast, endometrial and ovarian cancer. The Lancet. 4.24.1976

[2] DeLong, FR, et al. 1997 Effect on infant mortality of iodination of irrigation in water in a severely iodine-deficient area of China. Lancet. 350:771-773

[3] Foster, H. The iodine-selenium connection: Its possible roles in intelligence, cretinism, sudden infant death syndrome, breast cancer and multiple sclerosis. Medical Hypothesis. 40. 61-65. 1993

[4] WHO. IB1D3/27. 12 Nov. 1998

[5] WHO IBID 12 Nov. 1998

[6] Hollowell, JE et al. Iodine nutrition in the United States. Trends and public health implications: Iodine excretion data from National Health and Nutrition Examination Surveys I and III (1971-74 and 1988-94). J Clin Endocrinol Metab 83:3401-3408. 1998.

[7] Venkatesh, M, et al. Salt iodization for the elimination of iodine deficiency. 1995

[8] Abraham, G. Orthoidosupplementation: Iodine Sufficiency of the Whole Human Body. The Original Internist. December, 2002

[9] Dietary Reference Intakes (2001). Institute of Medicine

[10] Hollowell, JE et al. IBID. 1998.

[11] Pitman, JA. Changing normal values for thyroidal radioiodine uptake. NEJM. 1969;280:1431-34

[12] Abraham, G. The Concept of Orthoiodosupplementation and Its Clinical Implications. The Original Internist. June, 2004.

[13] Dunn, J. Editorial: What's happening to our iodine? J. of Clinical Endcrin. And Metab. Vol. 83, No. 10. 1998

[14] Vobecky, M. Effect of enhanced bromide intake on the concentration ratio I/Br in the rat thyroid gland. Bio. Trace Element Research, 43:509-513, 1994

[15] Abraham, G. Measurement of urinary iodide levels by ion-selective electrode: Improved sensitivity and specificity by chromatography on an ion-exchange resin. Optimox Research Info. IOD-03. 1.6.03

Chapter 3

Different Forms of Iodine

CHAPTER 3: DIFFERENT FORMS OF IODINE

Iodine is not very soluble in water. Jean Lugol, a French physician, was interested in substances that could treat infections and became very interested in iodine because it showed promise in this area. In 1829, Dr. Lugol found that potassium iodide added to water increased the solubility of iodine. Dr. Lugol began using a solution termed "Lugol's Iodine" that was a mixture of 5% iodine and 10% potassium iodide in water (see next page). Two drops of Lugol's solution (0.1ml) contains 5mg of iodine and 7.5mg of iodide. Iodide is the reduced form of iodine which contains an extra electron.

Dr. Lugol began treating many different infections with his solution and had great success. Dr. Lugol's recommended dose for a wide variety of problems was two drops per day of Lugol's solution. This provided 12.5mg of iodine, which is very similar to the physiologic dose of iodine for sufficiency of the entire body (see Chapter 7 for more information). Dr. Lugol's solution was widely available at apothecaries and was routinely prescribed for many different conditions.

Lugol's Iodine Solution

10% Potassium Iodide
5% Iodine
85% Distilled Water

IODIDE AND IODINE

As mentioned above, it is very difficult to get iodine into a solution that uses water as a solvent. Therefore, as Dr. Lugol discovered, using the reduced form of iodine (iodide) increased the solubility of iodine. In order to do this, iodine must first be reduced to iodide. For the science majors, this means that the molecule of iodine has gained an electron, which allows it to form a salt with certain elements like potassium and sodium. In the case of Lugol's solution, it is in the form of potassium iodide (10% in Lugol's solution). When there is a full complement of electrons in the iodine molecule, it is referred to as iodide.

It was thought that the intestinal tract could easily convert iodine to iodide, but research has shown this is not true.[1] Different tissues of the body respond to the different forms of iodine. The thyroid gland primarily utilizes iodide. To decrease the incidence of goiter, potassium iodide was added to table salt.

Donald, 49 years old, had Hashimoto's disease for ten years. Donald was found to be hypothyroid and to have many nutritional deficiencies. He was treated with Armour thyroid, vitamins and minerals, and diet changes (eliminating refined carbohydrates and trans-fatty acids). "I am definitely feeling much better with the thyroid hormone. I felt like I was dying before. But, I still don't feel like myself. I still have brain fog and some muscle aches," he stated. Iodine testing showed that Donald had iodine deficiency. He excreted only 35% of a challenge test of iodine (normal levels should be over 90%). Donald was initially treated with a form of iodide known as SSKI. He claimed, "I did not feel worse with the SSKI, I just did not feel better. I still had the brain fog while on it." Donald was switched to a mixture of iodine and iodide (Iodoral®) and he noticed a definite change. Iodoral® is a tablet form of Lugol's solution. "Within one week of starting the Iodoral®, my brain fog began to clear. I began sleeping better, my energy improved, and even my libido picked

61

up. I feel almost totally back to normal. Two months after taking 25mg of Iodoral® per day, his iodine test improved dramatically (94.4% secretion).

The breasts, on the other hand, primarily utilize iodine. Studies have shown that iodine deficiency can alter the structure and function of breast tissue.[2] This can include dysplasia and atypia that may be the forerunner for breast cancer. Animal studies have shown that iodide (the form of iodine that is present in iodized salt) is ineffective at reversing the pre-cancerous lesions of animal breast tissue, whereas iodine is much more effective.[3] Research has also shown that iodine, not iodide, will decrease lipoperoxidation of breast tissue.[4]

Lipoperoxidation is a chemical reaction that can cause damage to the lipids of the cell membrane and mitochondria. This can lead to many serious illnesses such as cancer and autoimmune disorders. Lipoperoxidation has been found to be elevated in breast tumors and animal breast tissue exposed to agents that promote cancer. Iodine decreases lipoperoxidation in the body. This will be more fully explored in Chapter 4.

Because different tissues concentrate different forms of iodine, using a supplement that contains both iodide and iodine is preferable to using a supplement that contains only one form. As mentioned above, the breasts concentrate iodine. The prostate gland concentrates iodine. The thyroid gland and the skin primarily concentrate iodide. Other tissues, including the kidneys, spleen, liver, blood, salivary glands, and intestines can concentrate either form. With different tissues responding to different forms of iodine, it would make common sense that a greater therapeutic benefit from iodine will be achieved by using a combination of iodine and iodide. My clinical experience has proven, beyond a doubt, that a combination of iodine/iodide (e.g., Lugol's or Iodoral®) is much more effective than an iodide only supplement (e.g., SSKI and most other liquid iodide formulations).

Leslie, a 43-year-old nurse, suffers with fibrocystic breast disease. "My breasts always hurt and before my period, I can't even stand to have a shirt on. The rubbing of clothing is excruciating," she said. Leslie had been to many doctors and was told to change her diet. She said, "Eliminating caffeine and chocolate did help somewhat, but I am still miserable." When I saw Leslie, she not only had a severe case of fibrocystic breast disease, she also had cysts on her ovaries. Leslie commented, "I kept thinking that there must be something wrong with me. Why would I be getting all of these cysts in my body?" On examination, Leslie had an enlarged thyroid gland and many signs of an underactive thyroid condition, including being very fatigued. Laboratory testing showed severe iodine deficiency with a 12% excretion on an iodine-challenge test (normal levels should be above 90%). Upon taking iodine (in the form of an iodine/iodide mixture—Iodoral®), Leslie noticed a dramatic improvement in her condition. "Within two weeks of taking iodine, I had more energy and within one month, my breast cysts began to fade. After taking the iodine for two months, my breasts were soft and the lumpiness was gone. It no longer hurts to wear clothing. It feels like a miracle," she said. The ovarian cysts Leslie had struggled with also resolved. Repeat testing of iodine levels showed a normal excretion rate on a challenge test (94% excretion). She was eventually treated with a holistic approach of vitamins, minerals, herbs, and natural hormones.

Leslie's case is not unique. The treatment of breast cysts with iodine has been reported for over 50 years. Most patients with breast cysts will significantly improve their condition with iodine supplementation. The next chapter contains more information on breast disease and iodine deficiency.

FINAL THOUGHTS

I have used various iodide preparations for years, with mixed success. Although preparations that solely contain iodide are effective for certain conditions such as sinusitis, there is clearly an advantage to using a combination of iodide and iodine together. The results that I have seen in my patients have convinced me that using a combination of iodide and iodine is a much more effective and appropriate treatment than using iodide alone.

Lugol's solution is an effective iodine supplement. The downside to Lugol's solution is the taste and the dosing of it. Lugol's has a distinct metallic taste that many people find offensive. In addition, the dosing of Lugol's can be inconsistent.

One drop may not be the same size each time it is measured. Therefore, I generally prefer a tablet form of iodine. The compliance with taking the medication is greater and the dosing is more consistent. The most important item to keep in mind with respect to an iodine supplement is that the supplement should have a combination of iodine and iodide present.

[1] Thrall, K. Distribution of iodine into blood components of the Sprague-Dawley rat differs with the chemical form administered. Fundamental and applied Toxicology. 15:75-81. 1990
[2] Eskin, B. Different tissue responses for iodine and iodide in rat thyroid and mammary glands. Biological Trace Element Research. Vol. 49, 1995
[3] Eskin, B. IBID. 1995
[4] Aceves, C. Is Iodine a gatekeeper of the integrity of the mammary gland? J. of Mammary Gland Biol. and Neoplasia. Vol. 10, No. 2. April 2005.

Chapter 4

Iodine, Breast Cancer and Fibrocystic Disease

CHAPTER 4: IODINE, BREAST CANCER AND FIBROCYSTIC DISEASE

Joan, a 60-year-old English teacher, was diagnosed with breast cancer in 1989. She refused conventional therapy and looked for other options. She found a holistic doctor who recommended that she take 2mg/day of iodine in addition to a regimen of vitamins and minerals. She was also diagnosed with hypothyroidism and treated with thyroid hormone. Over the next ten years, she felt well and continued to teach. The tumor metastasized in early 2005. Joan's tumor markers also increased and she felt very fatigued. She lost 25 pounds of weight by July 2005. "I felt like I was dying," she said. After she read of Dr. Abraham's research on iodine, she found a doctor to prescribe iodine for her. She increased the iodine dose from 2mg/day to 50-62.5mg/day using a tablet form of Lugol's (Iodoral®). As she increased the iodine, she was able to stop the thyroid hormone. After six weeks of taking the higher iodine dose, Joan had a PET scan. The PET scan showed that all of the existing tumors were disintegrating. The tumors were disintegrating from the center of the tumors after just 26 days of taking a higher dose of iodine. "I am so grateful for this information as it is surely saving my life," Joan claimed.

Joan's case is not unique. Iodine can cause tumors to shrink and necrose from the center. I have observed similar results with nodules and cysts in the thyroid, ovaries, and uterus after instituting orthoiodosupplementation.

This chapter will explore the relationship between iodine deficiency and disorders of the breast, including fibrocystic breast disease and breast cancer as well as other cancers. For over 60 years, it has been known that iodine concentrates in and is secreted by the mammary glands. The breasts are one of the body's main storage and utilization sites for iodine. An adequate iodine level is necessary for the development and maintenance of normal breast architecture. Milk from lactating breasts contains four times more of the ingested iodine than the amount taken up by the thyroid gland.[1]

Animal studies have shown conclusively that an iodine deficient state can alter the structure and function of the breasts. After my own research and study, I concur with several investigators that iodine deficiency is a causative factor in breast cancer and fibrocystic breast disease. I believe it is essential that women have their iodine levels tested, and if it is shown there is an iodine deficiency, iodine supplementation should be initiated.

The breasts are one of the body's main storage sites for iodine in the body. In an iodine-deficient state, the thyroid gland and the breasts will compete for what little iodine is available. Therefore, this will leave the thyroid gland and the breasts iodine depleted and can set the stage for illnesses such as goiter, hypothyroidism, autoimmune thyroid illness, breast illnesses including cancer, and cystic breast disease. In addition, other glandular tissues, such as the ovaries which contain the second highest concentration of iodine in the body, will also be depleted in an iodine deficient state.

IODINE: THE ANTICANCER AGENT

Iodine has many anticancer properties. Cancer cells, unlike normal cells, do not have a normal life cycle; they just keep dividing over and over. Normal cells have a life cycle, and when they eventually die, they are replaced with a new cell. This process of timed cellular death is known as apoptosis. Iodine has been shown to induce apoptosis (death) in breast and thyroid cancer cells. However, this apoptotic effect will be negated if a goitrogen is given.[2]

How does iodine provide this apoptotic effect? One mechanism may be the iodination of lipids. Lipids are fats that

71

make up our cell membranes throughout our body. Iodine can become incorporated into lipids (fats) inside the cell. These substances are known as iodolipids. When iodine is incorporated into the lipids, it helps to stabilize them and also helps each cell to maintain a normal life cycle.

Iodine has been shown to be a potent antioxidant even more effective than Vitamin E, phosphatidyl choline, and Vitamin C.[3] [4] [5] As with Vitamin C, iodine can function as both an antioxidant as well as an oxidant in the body. This dual effect makes it a strong anticancer agent. One of the best signs of health in the body is a balance between antioxidants and oxidants. Items like iodine and Vitamin C can help maintain that balance, and therefore, are some of the most powerful anti-cancer agents known.

Delores, an active 73-year-old woman, was diagnosed with breast cancer in 2003. She refused conventional therapy and wanted an alternative treatment. "Why would I do chemotherapy and radiation when the doctors told me that these treatments may not help? They could not give me good statistics that these treatments would prolong my life. When I asked them to help me find the cause of this illness, they just had a blank stare in their eyes. When I read about the relationship between iodine and breast cancer, I asked my doctor and he said, "There is enough iodine in salt". When I saw Delores, I measured her iodine and bromide levels as part of a study I was conducting on breast cancer patients. Her results are summarized on the next page.

72

Delores: Urinary Excretion of Iodide and Bromide Before and After Taking Iodine

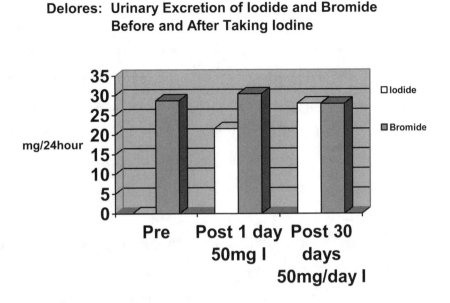

Delores' initial results show that she was excreting large amounts of the toxic halide bromide at the same time that her body was very deficient in iodine. After taking 50mg of iodine/iodide (Iodoral®), her bromide excretion increased and still was elevated after 30 days of taking iodine. At the same time that her body was absorbing iodine, it was also excreting the toxic halide bromine. Delores was treated with a holistic treatment program that included vitamins, minerals, and natural hormones in addition to other natural items to support her detoxification pathways. This included the use of Celtic Sea Salt®. The salt was utilized to help the body detoxify bromide. After three months on this program,

Delores felt significantly improved. "My energy level was so much better. I can now do ten times what I could do before," she said.

Delores had a repeat ultrasound 18 months after starting the iodine-based therapy and the radiologist reported on the ultrasound, "It would seem, therefore, that these malignancies have diminished considerably in size. The breast cancer appears considerably diminished when compared to previous ultrasound. Interval improvement is definitely seen."

There is a wealth of research showing the connection between iodine deficiency and breast cancer. We should be searching for underlying cause(s) of cancer and formulating a treatment program tailored to addressing the underlying cause(s). The "war" on breast cancer began 35 years ago. The progress in treating breast cancer with chemotherapy, surgery, and radiation has been dismal. Survival rates for breast cancer victims are virtually unchanged over the last 30 years, even with the use of mammograms, surgery, chemotherapy and radiation.

Iodine deficiency as well as other toxicities (especially the toxic halides bromine and fluoride) must be investigated. Perhaps rectifying iodine deficiency will be the missing piece of the puzzle to solving the riddle of breast cancer. Delores' case has been repeated over and over in my practice. I believe all women need to be evaluated for their iodine status before they reach the stage of breast cancer.

ESTROGENS AND IODINE: THE CONNECTION

This section will deal with the relationship between iodine and estrogens. Estrogens are a class of steroid hormones produced and secreted in both men and women. In men, most of the estrogen is produced in the adrenal glands, fat tissue, and liver. The amount of estrogen in men is ten times lower than it is in women.

In women, estrogens control female sexual development including promoting the growth and function of the female sexual organs such as the ovaries, uterus, and breasts. The ovaries produce most of the estrogen in women, with smaller amounts produced in the adrenal glands and the fat tissue.

DIFFERENT FORMS OF ESTROGEN

There are three major types of estrogen produced in the female body: estrone (E1), estradiol (E2), and estriol (E3). Estriol is a much weaker estrogen than either estrone or estradiol. Research has shown that estriol may be able to prevent breast cancer in mice.[6] Furthermore, estriol is less stimulating to breast tissue than either estradiol or estrone and may have a protective effect for breast cancer. My colleague, Jonathan Wright, M.D., measured the estrogen levels in healthy 20-40 year old women and found that estriol was produced at much larger amounts than either estrone or estradiol.[7] Estrogen replacement therapy has been promoted to help women with menopausal symptoms, osteoporosis, and other illnesses. Common sense would argue that to achieve the greatest benefit from estrogen replacement therapy, we should try to mimic the body's own production of estrogen. In other words, we should use the same proportions of estrone, estradiol, and estriol normally produced in the healthy body. Estrogen production in the body can be monitored by measuring the amounts of estrone, estradiol, and estriol that are present in biological fluid. When there are imbalances in estrogen production, such as lowered amounts of estriol and larger amounts of estrone and estradiol, problems such as fibrocystic breasts, cancer, and weight gain may develop.

Dr. Wright has reported compelling data that iodine, in the form of Lugol's solution (iodine, and iodide) can help maintain the correct balance of the three estrogens. Specifically, Dr. Wright has reported that Lugol's solution will help the body metabolize the estrogens to favor the safer form of estrogen—estriol. My experience has found the same results; the use of iodine helps to maintain a balanced estrogen ratio in favor of estriol.

For women, a balance of estrogens is vitally important for numerous bodily functions including ensuring optimal function of the brain, breast development, and lubrication of the skin. In addition, estrogen balance helps to ensure strong bones and helps to prevent cardiovascular disease. Imbalances in estrogen production are associated with weight gain, mood swings and disorders such as diabetes as well as cancer of the breast, ovary, and uterus. Estrogen balance is impossible to maintain when there is iodine deficiency present. For more information on the use of estrogens and other natural hormones, I refer the reader to my book, *The Miracle of Natural Hormones, 3rd Edition.*

IODINE DEFICIENCY AND THE BREASTS

Iodine deficiency has been shown to produce specific changes in the breast tissue of rats. Studies dating back nearly 40 years ago show that iodine deficiency in rats produces the exact precancerous changes seen in humans—dysplasia and hyperplasia.[8] [9] Furthermore, with long-term iodine depletion, more atypical changes in rat breast tissue occur.[10] This is the precursor to breast cancer.

Dr. Bernard Eskin, one of the world's foremost researchers on iodine and the breast, writes, "In all these studies, termination of dietary iodine restriction...results in a variable modest return toward the normal {breast} structure."[11]

Dr. Eskin has studied the effects of estrogen and iodine in rats. He has found that rats need an adequate level of iodine in order for estrogen to perform its normal function in breast tissue.[12]

It is known that the ovaries concentrate a large amount of iodine. After the thyroid, the ovaries have the second largest concentration of iodine in the body. Iodine deficiency produces changes in the ovarian production of estrogens as well as changes in the estrogen receptors of the breasts. In an iodine-deficient state, research has shown that ovarian estrogen production

77

increases, while estrogen receptors in the breast increase their sensitivity to estrogens.[13] [14] Both of these conditions will increase the risk of developing pathology of the breasts including breast cancer.

PUTTING IT ALL TOGETHOR: ESTROGEN AND IODINE AND THE CONNECTION TO CANCER

Iodine deficiency has many consequences. First, it causes estrogen production to increase. Iodine deficiency also leads to an increased sensitivity of breast tissue to estrogen. All of the above conditions will increase the chances of developing disease(s) of the breast including breast cancer. When you factor in our exposure to environmental estrogens, including xenoestrogens found in plastics, and pesticides, as well as meat and dairy products, it is no wonder that hormone-sensitive cancers like breast cancer have reached epidemic proportions. Research in animals has shown that the correction of iodine deficiency results in abnormal breast tissue changing back to normal breast tissue. My clinical experience has shown the same positive results occur with my human patients. This chapter will explore this concept in more detail.

FIBROCYSTIC BREAST DISEASE

Fibrocystic breast disease is a condition whereby the breasts have cysts that are usually painful to touch. Up to two-thirds of American women suffer from fibrocystic breast disease. In fibrocystic breast disease, the texture of the cysts can vary from soft to firm. Many times these cysts can change size and shape during the menstrual cycle, and they can cause discomfort premenstrually. Although fibrocystic breast disease is generally thought of as a benign condition, there are many physicians who feel that the abnormal breast architecture found in fibrocystic disease is a precursor for breast cancer, and this has been confirmed recently in various studies.[15][16][17]

Estrogens have been implicated as a causative factor for fibrocystic disease and breast cancer. In fact, one of the most common treatments in conventional medicine for fibrocystic disease is to use birth control pills to suppress the ovaries and lower the amount of circulating estrogen in the body.

As repeated hormonal cycles progress, oftentimes the fibrocystic changes in the breast will worsen. The breasts can become chronically inflamed and hardened. Many women suffer terribly with this illness.

Dietary factors can also worsen fibrocystic breast disease. Caffeine and foods that contain trans-fatty acids can exacerbate fibrocystic breast disease. Eliminating caffeine and eating foods rich in healthy fats, including essential fatty acids, will help alleviate many of the complaints of fibrocystic breast disease.

Also, vitamin and mineral supplementation can alleviate this condition. Vitamin E and Vitamin A have both been shown in studies to improve fibrocystic breasts.

Iodine has also been shown to be extremely effective in treating and preventing fibrocystic breasts.[18] In fact, iodine has been the most researched mineral in treating fibrocystic breast disease.

MaryAnn, age 45, works as a nurse at a local hospital. MaryAnn suffered from fibrocystic breast disease for over 15 years. She said, "My breasts feel like two rocks. I can't do aerobics or exercise heavily because the bouncing causes tremendous pain." MaryAnn was going to a specialized cystic breast clinic at the University of Michigan. Frequently, she was having breast cysts drained, only to have them reappear a short time later. Dietary changes, including removing the caffeine did help somewhat. MaryAnn was so miserable she was contemplating a mastectomy. MaryAnn was found to be severely iodine deficient (iodine challenge test showed 27% excretion with normal levels >90%). She was treated with Iodoral® 50mg per day and within one month had a dramatic change in her condition. She called me on the phone and reported, "Dr. Brownstein, I was at the University of Michigan clinic yesterday and the doctor told me he thought my breasts weren't mine. The two rocks I had are now soft and normal feeling. All of the cysts are gone and all of the pain is gone. This has been a miracle for me. I can't believe one nutrient could have such a positive impact on my life."

Darlene, at age 39, suffered from fibrocystic breast disease for over five years. "Sometimes I am absolutely miserable. I

80

cannot stand anything touching my breasts. It feels like there is a tourniquet around them," she said. Darlene's symptoms would get worse around her menses. She said, "My husband knows not to get within five feet of me. If I bump into anything, I feel like crying." Darlene was told to alter her diet and give up caffeine and chocolate, which did help her symptoms. "The change in the diet did help, but I was still miserable," she claimed. When I checked Darlene's iodine levels, her iodine-loading tests showed a 50% excretion (normal is 90%). After two weeks of supplementing with an iodine/iodide combination (Iodoral®), Darlene's condition rapidly improved. "I just woke up one morning and I wasn't in pain. I could not believe it. I feel like I have been given my life back," she said. In addition, the iodine significantly improved her energy and mood levels. Darlene says, "I can't believe how much better I feel."

MaryAnn and Darlene's cases are typical of many with fibrocystic breast disease. Usually, the improvement in fibrocystic symptoms occurs rapidly when there is an iodine-deficient state present.

THYROID DISEASE, IODINE, AND CANCER

For well over 100 years, iodine deficiency has been associated with a swelling of the thyroid or goiter — see Chapter 2 for more information. Goiter has also been associated with cancers of the breast, stomach, esophagus, ovaries, and uterus.[19] [20] [21] My colleague, Jorge Flechas, M.D., reports a "definite increase in the incidence of breast cancer, stomach cancer, ovarian cancer, and thyroid cancer with the presence of iodine deficiency."[22] I have seen similar results in my practice.

BREAST CANCER AND HYPOTHYROIDISM

The relationship between hypothyroidism and breast cancer has been reported for over 100 years. In fact, the first reported connection between these two illnesses was mentioned in 1896. Although there has not been a consensus opinion on the relationship between breast cancer and hypothyroidism, many researchers feel there is a direct connection.

Researchers have found that hypothyroidism is much more common in women with breast cancer.[23][24] Other researchers have found that the use of thyroid hormones may cause a higher incidence of breast cancer.[25] Although there has been a great controversy in medicine on verifying the relationship between hypothyroidism and breast cancer, my experience has shown that there is a connection.

It is known that hypothyroidism predisposes one to a poorly functioning immune system. This can set the stage for serious illnesses such as cancer. One would think that the treatment of hypothyroidism with thyroid hormone would improve the condition of breast cancer, since it should improve the functioning of the immune system. However, this has not been shown to be the case in some studies. In fact, some studies point to an exacerbation of breast cancer when thyroid hormones are used to treat a hypothyroid condition.

WHY WOULD THE TREATMENT OF HYPOTHYROIDISM RESULT IN AN INCREASED RISK OF BREAST CANCER? THE IODINE CONNECTION.

When hypothyroidism is present, the body is in a hypometabolic state. In other words, all bodily functions slow down and the consequences of this state include cold extremities, dry skin, fatigue, brain fog and weight gain. When thyroid hormone is given, it results in an increased metabolic state which reverses all of the above conditions.

ATP is the body's "high octane" energy source. Thyroid hormone utilizes ATP to increase the body's metabolic rate. This increased metabolism helps the body produce more heat, lose weight, overcome fatigue, etc. If thyroid hormone is given to an iodine-deficient patient, the increased metabolic rate due to thyroid hormone will actually increase the body's need for iodine as well as decreasing the ability of the cells of the body to concentrate iodine.

Iodine uptake by the cells is an energy dependent process which requires ATP. Thyroid hormones use the energy available for the synthesis of ATP to produce heat. This effect lowers the available ATP for cellular uptake of iodine by the target cells. If there are lowered ATP levels in the body, the target cells have a more difficult time concentrating iodine.

Finally, if a hypothyroid condition is treated with thyroid hormone and there is also iodine deficiency present, the use of thyroid hormone will exacerbate an iodine-deficient condition.

The only logical explanation that ties the treatment of hypothyroidism with an increased risk of developing breast cancer would be the presence of an iodine deficiency.

In simpler terms, thyroid hormones introduced into the body will raise the body's need for iodine. The breasts, like the thyroid gland, have an advanced system for absorbing and storing iodine. When there is iodine deficiency, the breast and the thyroid gland enlarge to compensate for that deficiency. In both cases, iodine deficiency induces hyperplasia, which is a precancerous lesion. This will set the stage for thyroid and breast diseases, including cancer of the thyroid gland and the breasts.

If iodine deficiency is present, the use of thyroid hormone supplementation without first correcting (or simultaneously correcting) the iodine deficit will exacerbate the body's deficit of iodine. The result of this can be an increase in disorders caused by iodine deficiency such as cancers of the breast and thyroid.

THE BREASTS AND IODINE

The therapeutic use of iodine in treating breast cancer was first described in the medical literature in 1896.[26] There is a direct relationship between breast cancer (as well as goiter) and regions

84

of the world where iodine deficiency is prevalent. Countries such as Japan and Iceland have higher intakes of iodine and lower rates of goiter and breast cancer. On the other hand, countries such as the United States, Mexico and Thailand have lower iodine intake and higher incidences of both breast cancer and goiter.[27] Some countries such as Poland, Switzerland, Australia and Russia have been found to have high rates of breast cancer associated with localized pockets of iodine deficiency. In the United States, a correlation has been found between higher mortality rates from breast cancer and areas of iodine deficiency (e.g., Great Lakes region).[28]

Cathy, 49 years old, was diagnosed with breast cancer one year ago. She said, "I was devastated. I thought I took good care of myself and my life was shattered. When I asked the surgeon, 'How did I get it?' He answered, 'I don't know'. His only concern was doing surgery and getting me ready for chemotherapy. I was not satisfied with that." Cathy did elect to have a bilateral mastectomy and chemotherapy, but still searched for why this may have happened to her. When I examined Cathy, I found her to have a serum iodine level below the detection limits as well as having a very low iodine loading test—22% (normal > 90%). In treating her with iodine/iodide (Iodoral®), she noticed an immediate improvement in her overall health. "I was having fatigue and leg cramps. The fatigue was debilitating. I felt like an old woman," she said. Three weeks after starting the iodine, both conditions improved dramatically. "It was a miracle. The leg cramps and leg pains melted away but, more importantly, the fatigue left. My brain started functioning again, and I began to feel like my old self. Even my friends began asking me what I was taking, since I looked so much better," she said.

Iodine was found to have a suppressive effect on the development and the size of mammary tumors in rats.[29] This suppressive effect was enhanced with the use of progesterone. The enhancement of iodine uptake with progesterone has also been found in other tissue including the uterus and the ovary.[30] These studies prove that the optimal use of iodine is best undertaken as part of a comprehensive holistic treatment program, which emphasizes balancing the hormonal system as well as correcting nutrient deficits. For more information, I refer the reader to my book, *The Miracle of Natural Hormones, 3ʳᵈ Edition.*

THE BREASTS AND TOXIC HALIDES: IS THERE AN ASSOCIATION WITH BREAST CANCER?

The halides are a group of elements that share a similar size and shape. Chapter 5 will cover this topic in much more detail. Fluoride, bromine, iodine, chlorine and astatine make up this family. Iodine is the only halide that has therapeutic effects in the body.

Bromide is a toxic element that has a chemical structure very similar to iodine. This similarity can cause bromine to bind to iodine receptors and possibly interfere with iodine transport in the body. Bromine is found in many food items such as bakery products, and some sodas, as well as many prescription items. In addition, bromine is found in many fire-retardant chemicals added to furniture, carpets, etc. Crops are sprayed with bromine as a fumigant for agriculture. When there is iodine deficiency present, bromine toxicity will be exacerbated.

Fluoride is put in the water supply, toothpaste, and many drinks as a preventive measure against dental caries. There is little evidence to support the idea that fluoride prevents cavities. Furthermore, there is much research that shows that fluoride (in the amounts ingested by drinking fluoridated water) can cause dental fluorosis, hip fractures, bone cancer, and other negative effects. Fluoride toxicity will be covered in more detail in Chapter 5.

I undertook a study in my office to look at the difference in iodine, fluoride, and bromine levels in eight women with breast cancer versus ten women without breast cancer. Please refer to Chapter 5 for a further discussion of this study and the results.

This study showed that all of the women tested--those with breast cancer as well as those without breast cancer--had low iodine levels. Those women with breast cancer were found to have much larger amounts of the toxic halides bromine and fluoride as compared to the women without breast cancer. The toxicity of bromine and fluoride are exacerbated in an iodine-deficient state.

Perhaps the reason we have an epidemic of breast cancer is not only due to iodine deficiency, but also to the toxicity of halogens fluoride and bromine which inhibit iodine uptake by the tissues of the body. Effective breast cancer therapies will not be realized until the causative factors of breast cancer (i.e., toxins) are more thoroughly studied.

THE JAPANESE: A POPULATION WITH A HIGH IODINE INTAKE AND A LOW RATE OF BREAST DISEASE AND GOITER

It has been estimated that the mainland Japanese ingest approximately 13.8mg of iodine per day, which is over 100 times the RDA.[31] Japanese from the coastal areas ingest more iodine than the average inland Japanese consume. The mainland Japanese receive much of their iodine from seaweed, which is known to concentrate iodine.

What is the effect of ingesting this larger amount of iodine? The Japanese, who consume a large amount of iodine by U.S. RDA standards, have remarkably lower levels of breast, endometrial, and ovarian cancers. In addition, there is a significantly lower amount of fibrocystic breast disease in Japanese women who consume the larger amount of iodine. Over 30 years ago, research showed that Japanese women who move to the United States have a higher rate and mortality of breast, endometrial, and ovarian cancer as compared to mainland Japanese women.[32] I believe this increase in mortality of Japanese women is due to falling iodine levels.

It has been known for over 50 years that there is an association between breast cancer and iodine levels. There have been many articles written in medical literature pointing towards a direct relationship between low iodine levels and the development of breast cancer in various regions of the world, including the United States.[33] [34]

Joyce, 52 years old, was diagnosed with breast cancer two years ago. "I thought I was in great shape. I used to exercise, and I watched what I ate. When I was diagnosed with breast cancer, I was devastated," she said. Joyce did not want to undergo chemotherapy and radiation. Joyce claimed, "I did not have a chemotherapy and radiation deficiency. I have done a lot of reading on breast cancer, and I was worried about the side effects from the chemotherapy and radiation. I wanted to search for an underlying cause and find a treatment for that." Joyce had a long history of fibrocystic breast disease and dense breasts on a mammogram. My initial examination and laboratory workup of Joyce revealed an enlarged thyroid gland (i.e., goiter). Laboratory tests showed evidence of a poorly functioning immune system (low natural killer cells and low immunoglobulin levels as well as a low white blood cell count). An iodine-loading test showed Joyce was extremely low (12% excretion with normal levels >90%). Joyce was treated with a combination of iodine/iodide (Iodoral®) four pills per day (50mg of iodide/iodine) for three months. After three months, her iodine-loading test improved to normal and her dose of iodine was lowered to two pills per day (25mg). During that time, Joyce noticed an improvement in her energy and overall better health. "I felt wonderful once I started taking iodine. My energy level zoomed up and my metabolism increased. All my friends started asking me what I was doing, since I looked so much better," she said. Joyce was also treated holistically with a detoxification program and given vitamins and minerals. Her laboratory markers all improved as well. Her doctors felt the changes in her breasts. "My doctor told me that my breast tissue felt much softer. He said that my breasts felt much healthier," she claimed. With her improved laboratory markers, I feel Joyce will have a better chance to overcome her illness. Was iodine deficiency the underlying cause of her cancer? I don't have the definitive answer to that question, but an iodine-deficient state will not only set the stage for breast illness such as cancer to develop, it will make it extremely difficult for the body to overcome such illnesses.

IODINE DEFICIENCY AND PROSTATE CANCER

Although the research is not as complete as it is for breast cancer, I believe the cause(s) of prostate cancer in men is similar to the cause(s) of breast cancer in women. Japanese men have much lower rates of prostate cancer than American men. Japanese men that move to the United States have a higher rate of prostate cancer than mainland Japanese. This analogy is similar to the increased incidence of breast cancer in Japanese women who move to the United States. I believe iodine deficiency is the link (or at least one of the links) and is responsible for the increased risk of prostate cancer. Mainland Japanese men have a much lower prostate cancer mortality rate than American men because of their higher iodine intake. When iodine levels fall, the rates of prostate cancer will begin to increase. I believe future research needs to be directed in this area.

ANIMALS IN AN IODINE DEFICIENT STATE WILL DEVELOP BREAST CANCER

Animal research has shown that in an iodine deficient state, whether by diet or drug therapy, animal breast tissue will show signs of developing breast cancer. The longer the animals are maintained in an iodine deficient state, the more likely their breast tissue will become cancerous.[35] [36] Researchers have concluded, "It thus appears that maintenance of the optimum structure and function of the breasts requires the presence of continuous and specific amounts of iodine."[37] The use of estrogens causes worsening changes in the breast tissue, with additional signs of cancer being present upon examination of tissue.[38] In fact, iodine deficiency is found to enhance the response of animal breast tissue to estrogen injections.[39] Iodine deficiency, coupled with exogenous estrogens from the diet (e.g., hormones fed to animals) or chemicals in the environment (e.g., phthalates from plastics), could explain the epidemic of breast cancer that is occurring in this

91

country (as well as in many other western countries).

However, there is hope. Iodine deficiency disorders can easily be corrected with the addition of iodine to the diet. The correction of iodine deficiency in animals results in changing their breast tissue to assume a more normal architecture.

Many other tissues in the body utilize iodine besides the thyroid gland and the breasts. The prostate gland, gastrointestinal tract, salivary glands, bones, connective tissues, and the fluids of almost the entire body utilize iodine. These different tissues of the body all have developed iodine-trapping mechanisms to effectively extract iodine from dietary sources. The breasts have an efficient method of acquiring iodine from the diet.[40] The thyroid gland's need for iodine will ensure that it has the "first pick" of iodine which, in a deficient state may mean that other tissues of the body can show signs of severe deficiencies.

The iodization of salt was introduced solely to decrease the rate of goiter and mental retardation. It has decreased the prevalence of goiter, but it has not been enough to affect the rate of breast disease. In fact, areas of the world with the lowest iodine intakes have been found to have very high rates of breast cancer.

In the United States, the area known as the "goiter belt", which borders the Great Lakes, not only has the highest mortality rate from breast cancer it also has extremely low iodine levels in the soil. This would point to a direct relationship between iodine levels and development of and mortality from breast cancer.

When iodine is ingested or injected, there are two major areas of the body that take up iodine: the thyroid gland and the extra-thyroidal tissue. Researchers have estimated that approximately 8mg of iodine is taken up by the extra-thyroidal tissue (while 6mg is taken up by the thyroid).[41][42] The breasts are the largest consumers of extra-thyroidal iodine. Estimates are that the breasts need approximately 5mg of iodine per day in a 50kg (110lb) woman.[43][44][45] A larger woman (or a woman with larger breasts) would have a greater amount of iodine concentrated in the breasts. Since men have smaller breasts than women, their iodine needs are lower.

In a state of iodine deficiency, the body's major storage of iodine occurs in the thyroid gland. When the body becomes iodine sufficient, the thyroid gland will contain 50mg of iodine out of a total body iodine of 1,500mg-2,000mg.[46][47] At iodine sufficiency, the largest amounts of iodine are found in fat tissue and muscle (striated) tissue. If obesity is present, the body's need for iodine increases as the fat cells of the body would require more iodine.

As previously mentioned, women's breasts are major sites for iodine storage. Maintaining adequate iodine levels is necessary to ensure an adequately functioning thyroid gland and normal breast architecture. I believe it will also lower the incidence of breast cancer and help women overcome breast cancer.

It is well known that thyroid illnesses, including goiter and autoimmune thyroid disorders, strike women at much larger percentages than they strike men. One reason may be that a

93

woman, having more breast tissue than a man, requires a higher iodine intake than a man. In an iodine deficient state, a woman will show earlier signs and more severe signs of iodine deficiency than a man in a similar deficient state.

OTHER TISSUE REQUIREMENTS FOR IODINE

All of the glands of the body depend on adequate iodine levels to function optimally. Animal studies have shown problems with the adrenal glands[48], the thymus gland[49], the ovaries[50], the hypothalamus and pituitary axis[51], as well as the entire endocrine system, when there is an iodine deficient state. In fact, the ovaries have the second highest concentration of iodine in the body next to the thyroid gland. An iodine deficient state will lead to an imbalanced hormonal system. It is impossible to have a balanced hormonal system without ensuring an adequate iodine intake.

Dr. Guy Abraham, one of the world's leading researchers on iodine, has shown that the required daily intake of iodine necessary for maintaining iodine sufficiency for the whole body is at least 13mg per day.[52]

At sufficiency, the thyroid gland holds a total of approximately 50mg of iodine. The thyroid gland needs approximately 6mg/day of iodine for sufficiency. The breasts need at least 5mg of iodine; that leaves 2mg (13mg-11mg) of iodine for the rest of the body. This 2mg is still well above the RDA (14x the RDA) of 150ug/day of iodine. Either way, this would explain why the RDA for iodine is inadequate and why it is necessary not only

94

to get your iodine levels evaluated but, more importantly, to supplement with the correct amount and form of iodine.

FINAL THOUGHTS

The connection between iodine deficiency and breast cancer as well as fibrocystic breast disease is strong. Breast cancer (like prostate cancer) is occurring at epidemic rates—currently one in seven women are afflicted. Prostate cancer affects one in three men. Although there are numerous reasons for the development of cancer, the research is clear; iodine deficiency is a major piece of the puzzle. Iodine deficiency has also been associated with other cancers including ovarian, uterine, and thyroid cancer. It is imperative to have your iodine level checked and supplemented with the correct form of iodine when there is iodine deficiency present as part of an anti-cancer program.

[1] Bretthauer,E. Milk transfer comparisons of different chemical forms of radioiodine. Health Physics. 1972.22:257

[2] Vitale, M. Iodide excess induces apoptosis in thyroid cells through a p53-independent mechanism involving oxidative stress. Endocrin. 141. 2000.

[3] Smyth, P. Role of iodine in antioxidant defense in thyroid and breast disease. Biofactors. 19. 2003

[4] Tseng, Y.L. Iodothyronines: Oxidative deiodination by hemoglobin and inhibition of lipid peroxidation. Lipds. 19. 1984

[5] Winkler, R. Effects of iodide on total antioxidant status of human serum. Cell Biochem. Funct. 18. 2000.

[6] Lemon, H. Reduced estriol excretion in patients with breast cancer prior to endocrine therapy. JAMA. 196;1128-1136. 1966.

[7] Wright, Jonathan. Presented at ACAM. November, 2005. Anaheim, CA.

[8] Eskin, B. Mammary gland dysplasia. JAMA. 200. 1967

[9] Aquino, T. Arch. Pathology. 94, 270

[10] Krouse, T. Proc. Amer. Ass. Ca. Res. 18, 1977

[11] Eskin, B. Iodine and Mammary Cancer. Adv. In Exp. Medicine and Biology. Vol. 91. 1977

[12] Eskin, B. IBID. 1977

[13] Slebodzinski, A.B. Ovarian iodide uptake and triiodothyronine generation in follicular fluid. The enigma of the thyroid ovary interaction. Domest. Anim. Endocrinol. 29(1):97-103, July 2005

[14] Siiteri, P. Increased availability of serum estrogens in breast cancer, a new hypothesis. In Hormones and Breast Cancer. Banbury Repot No. 8. Cold Spring Harbour Laboratories, 1981

[15] Eskin, B., et al. Iodine metabolism and breast cancer. Trans. New York, Acad. of Sciences. 32:911-947, 1970

[16] Wang, J., Effects of tamoxifen on benign breast disease in women at high risk for breast cancer. J. Natl. Cancer Inst., 95 (4):202-207, 2003

[17] Bartow, S.A., et. al. Fibrocystic disease: A continuing enigma. Pathol. Annu. 1982: 17:93-111

[18] Ghent, W., et al. Iodine Replacement in Fibrocystic Disease of the Breast. Can.J. Surg. 36: 453-460, 1993

[19] Stadel, VV. Dietary iodine and risk of breast, endometrial and ovarian cancer. Lancet. 1976;1:890-891.

[20] Talamini, R. Selected medical conditions and risk of breast cancer. British J. of Cancer. 1997;75(11):1699-1703

[21] Venturi, S. Role of iodine in evolution and carcinogenesis of thyroid, breast and stomach. Adv. Clin. Path. 2000;4:11-17

[22] Flechas, J. Orthoiodosupplementation in a primary care practice. The Original Internist. 12(2):89-96, 2005.

[23] Smyth, P.P.A. Thyroid disease and breast cancer. J.Endocr. Invest. 16:396. 1993

[24] Perry, M. Thryoid function in patients with breast cancer. Ann. Roy. Coll. Surg. Engl. 60, 1978

[25] Chandrakant, C. Breast cancer relationship to thyroid supplements for hypothyroidism. JAMA. Vol. 236, No. 10. 9.6.1976.

[26] Beatson, G. Adjuvant use of thyroid extract in breast cancer. Lancet 104:no.2, pg. 162, 1896

[27] Finley, J.W., et all. Breast cancer and thyroid disease. Quart. Rev. Surg. Obstet. and Gyn. 1960 17: 139

[28] Eskin, B.A. Iodine and mammary cancer. Tans. N.Y. Acad. of Sciences. 1970

[29] Funaltashi, H. Suppressive effect of iodine on DM AA-induced breast cacner in rat. J. Surg. Oncol. 1996;61

[30] Brown-Grant, K. The sites of iodide concentration in the oviduct and the uterus of the rat. J. Endocrin. 1972;53.

[31] Abraham, G.E., et al. Orthoiodosupplementation: Iodine sufficiency of the whole shuman body. The Original Internist, 9:30-41, 2002

[32] Stadel, B. Dietary iodine and risk of breast, endometrial and ovarian cancer. Lancet. 4.24. 1976

[33] Bogardus, aG. Surgery. 1960, 49, 461.

[34] Finley, J. rev. Obstet. Gynec. 1960, 49, 17.

[35] Eskin, B.A. Iodine and mammary cancer. Tans. N.Y. Acad. of Sciences. 1970

[36] Drouse, T. Age-related changes in iodine-blocked. Proc. Amer. Ass. Ca. res. 18. 1977

[37] Eskin, B.A. Iodine and mammary cancer. Tans. N.Y. Acad. of Sciences. 1970

[38] Eskin, B.A. Mammary gland dysplasia in iodine deficiency. JAMA. 5.22.1967

[39] Eskin, B.A. IBID. 1967

[40] Eskin, B.A., et al. Human Breast Uptake of Radioactive Iodine. OB-GYN, 44:398-402, 1974

[41] Berson, S.A., et al. Quantitative aspects of iodine metabolism. The exchangeable organic iodine pool and the rates of thyroidal secretion, peripheral degradation and fecal excretion of endogenously synthesized organically bound iodine. J. Clin. Ivest, 33:1533-1552. 1954

[42] Abraham, G., et al. IBID. 2002

[43] Eskin, B., et al. Mammary Gland Dysplasia in Iodine Deficiency, JAMA, 200: 115-119, 1967.

[44] Eskin, B., etal. Iodine metabolism and Breast cancer. Tans. New York. Acad. Of sciences, 32: 911-947, 1970

[45] Abraham, G. IBID. 20025

[46] Koutras, D.A., et al. Effect of small iodine supplement on thyroid function in normal individuals. J. Clin. Endocr. 24:857-862, 1964

[47] Abraham, G., et al. Orthoiodosupplementation: Iodine sufficiency of the whole human body. Original Internist. December, 2002.

[48] Nolan, L.A., et al. Chronic Iodine deprivation attenuates stress-induced and diurnal variation in corticosterone secretion in female Wistar rats. J. Neuroend. 2000. Dec;12(12);1149-59

[49] Rodzaevskaia, E.B., et al. Age-dependent thymus involution in experimental iodine deficiency. Arkh. Patol. 2002 Mar-Apr;64(2):13-6

[50] Rodzaevskaia, E.B. Morphological impairment of oogenesis in experimental iodine-dependent thyroid transformation. Arkh. Patol. 2002. Mar-Apr; 64(2):10-3

[51] Nolan, et al. IBID. 2000

[52] Abraham, G. IBID. 2002

Chapter 5

Iodine and Toxic Halogens: Bromide and Fluoride

CHAPTER 5: IODINE AND THE TOXIC HALOGENS: BROMIDE AND FLUORIDE

Iodine is part of a class of elements known as the halogens. The halogens are a family of elements that form similar salt-like compounds in combination with sodium and most metals. The halogens are bromine, chlorine, fluorine, iodine, and astatine. The halogens, for chemistry enthusiasts, are found in group VIIa of the periodic table.

BROMINE

Bromine was discovered in 1826. Bromide, (the reduced form of bromine), is rapidly absorbed in the intestinal tract. Bromine lies just above iodine in the periodic table. Because the size and weight of bromine is very close to iodine, these two items can compete with one another for binding in the body, especially in the thyroid gland. Bromine, being a similar size and shape, has the ability to bind to iodine receptors in the body.

However, bromine should be considered to be a toxic element to the body and should be avoided. When bromide binds to the thyroid gland, it is not only a toxic element, it worsens an iodine deficient problem. Bromine is very slowly eliminated from the body.

Bromine intoxication (i.e., bromism) has been shown to cause delirium, psychomotor retardation, schizophrenia, and hallucination.[1] Subjects who ingest enough bromide feel dull and apathetic and have difficulty concentrating.[2] Bromide can also cause severe depression, headaches, and irritability. It is unclear how much bromide must be absorbed before symptoms of bromism become apparent. Recent research has demonstrated that symptoms of bromide toxicity can be present even with low levels of bromide in the diet.[3]

Bromine (or its reduced form—bromide) is used as an antibacterial agent for pools and hot tubs. It is still used as a fumigant for agriculture. Crops sprayed with bromide have been found to have elevated bromide levels.[4] Bromide is also used as a fumigant for termites and other pests. In 1981, 6.3 million pounds of bromide were used in California. By 1991, 18.7 million pounds were used in California.[5] Toxicity of bromine has been reported from the ingestion of some carbonated drinks (e.g., Mountain Dew, AMP Energy Drink, some Gatorade products), which contain brominated vegetable oils.[6]

Bromine used to be present in many common over-the-counter medications. It is still used today in many prescription medicines. Over 150 years ago, bromine was used extensively in medicine as a sedative as well as a remedy for seizures. Due to the toxicity of bromine, it has been phased out of many medicines. However, bromine still can be found in some medicines including those that treat asthma, and bowel and bladder dysfunction (see table below).

Some Currently Used Bromide-Containing Medications	
Medicine	**Indication**
Atrovent Inhaler	Breathing Difficulties
Atrovent Nasal Spray	Breathing Difficulties
Ipratropium Nasal Spray	Breathing Difficulties
Pro-Panthine	Bladder Dysfunction
Pyridostigmine bromide	Antidote for Nerve Gas
Spiriva Handihaler	Breathing Difficulties

I believe all medicines (as well as foods) that contain bromide need to be avoided. It is lunacy to use bromine in any form (either bromine or bromide) as a medicine. Animal studies have shown that bromide intake can adversely affect the accumulation of iodide in the thyroid and the skin.[7] Research has also shown that a high bromide intake would result in iodide being eliminated from the thyroid gland and being replaced by bromide.[8] In addition, animal studies have shown that the ingestion of bromide can cause hypothyroidism.[9] When there is iodine deficiency present, the toxicity of bromide is accelerated. Therefore, maintaining adequate iodine levels is essential when you live in an environment that provides exposure to bromide.

BROMINE ADDED TO BAKERY PRODUCTS

In the early 1960's, iodine was used in the manufacturing process of bakery products, including bread, as an anti-caking agent. One slice of bread contained up to 150ug of iodine, which was the RDA for iodine. In 1965, The National Institute of Health reported that the average iodine intake from bakery products was 726ug of iodine per day.[10] Some researchers felt that this amount of iodine could cause problems with the thyroid gland. Due to the erroneous concern of getting too much iodine from bakery products, iodine was replaced with bromine in the 1980's.[11]

This was a tremendous mistake. As can be seen from previous chapters, the amount of iodine in the bakery products was not even close to approaching a toxic level. The replacement of iodine by bromine not only increased the incidence of iodine deficiency, it also increased the levels of bromine in the population.

Bromine is a toxic element and has no place for ingestion in man. Bromine is considered a goitrogen, which is a chemical that causes a goiter of the thyroid gland. Bromine interferes with iodide uptake and utilization in the thyroid gland.[12] [13] There is no reason to use bromine in a medication and certainly no reason to use bromine in a common food source.

The substitution of bromine for iodine in bakery products is certainly a large part of the declining iodine levels in the United States. From 1971 until 2000, the National Health and Nutrition Survey (NHANES) showed iodine levels have declined 50% in the United States.[14] The authors of this study claim, "This reduction may be due, in part, to changes in food production."[15] No doubt, these authors must be referring to the substitution of bromine for iodine.

The effects of iodine on the body have been reviewed in previous chapters (see Chapter 2). The thyroid gland, the breasts, the salivary glands, etc., all have iodine receptor sites. The consequence of bromine binding to the iodine receptors in these tissues is disastrous. In the case of the thyroid gland, thyroid hormone production will be inhibited. The ingestion of bromine in an iodine-deficient state will further exacerbate thyroid illness.

HOW DO YOU LOWER BROMINE LEVELS?

Due to the addition of bromide in many food and drug sources (mentioned above), I believe that our bodies have bromide toxicity, which is further exacerbated by iodine deficiency. In order to improve one's endocrine and immune system, a practical way of helping the body detoxify from bromine must be found.

There are simple ways of lowering the levels of bromine in the body. Primarily, we must stop ingesting bromide-containing food and medicines. That means eating organic food, grown without pesticides. Also, it means limiting bakery products that contain bromine.

However, once bromide is absorbed, it binds tightly to the iodine receptors in the body. In addition, bromine can bind to the transport cells for iodine (sodium-iodide symporter—NIS) and damage the transporter cells. The oxidized form of bromide-bromine- is stored in the fat tissues. Taking iodine in physiologic doses can help to competitively inhibit the binding of bromine. Also, iodine supplementation allows the body to detoxify itself from bromine, while retaining iodine.

Research has shown that bromide competes with iodide for absorption and uptake in the body.[16] Dr. Guy Abraham, a researcher on iodine writes, "Therefore, increasing iodide intake should lower bromide levels in the thyroid preventing and reversing its thyrotoxic and goitrogenic effects."[17] The use of iodine will also cause bromine to be released from other tissues in the body in addition to the thyroid. Dr. Abraham showed that increasing the intake of iodine would additionally increase the urinary excretion of other toxic halides.[18] In fact, Dr. Abraham has shown that iodine supplementation can result "in the whole body being detoxified" from the toxic elements bromide and fluoride. Research done in my office verified this statement from Dr. Abraham.

Salt can also help with the removal of bromide. The chloride in salt is part of the halide family (iodide, chloride, fluoride and bromine). Chloride can competitively inhibit bromide and help the kidneys excrete bromide.[19] [20] [21] In fact, nearly 100 years ago, "salting the bromide out" was used in medicine to help lower bromine toxicity.

A low-salt diet will exacerbate bromine toxicity. When rats are subjected to a low-salt diet, the half-life of bromine is prolonged 833% as compared to rats given a normal salt diet.[22] Unrefined salt is an effective tool to help lower bromine levels in the body. For more information on salt, including more detailed information on salt and detoxification, I refer the reader to my book, ***Salt Your Way to Health.***

My clinical experience with the use of iodine has shown that the detoxifying effect of iodine supplementation translates into an improved immune system, a balanced hormonal system and more importantly, improvement in my patients' overall health.

Ellen is a 39 year-old school teacher. Ellen had a history of hypothyroidism and was being treated with thyroid hormone.

Though Ellen felt better on thyroid hormone, she still felt fatigued and suffered from headaches. The thyroid hormone made her symptoms improve by approximately 50%. When Ellen was checked for iodine, her loading test was low at 46% excretion (normal >90% excretion). Ellen was also checked for bromide excretion and was found to be excreting a large amount of bromine—131.5mg/24 hours (normal should be less than 5mg/24 hours). Upon being placed on 50mg of iodine/iodide (Iodoral®), her remaining symptoms initially worsened. "I felt more fatigued and my headaches increased in frequency," she said. I told Ellen that she was going through a detoxification process. The iodine was helping her body excrete large amounts of bromide. During a detoxification process, the body's detoxification systems need proper support to ensure the toxic chemicals can be safely released without harming the body's tissues. I told Ellen to take large amounts of Vitamin C—10,000mg/day, as Vitamin C helps all of the body's detoxification pathways function more effectively. Furthermore, I placed Ellen on 10gm of unrefined sea salt per day—Celtic Sea Salt®. The unrefined salt has chloride which can assist in the body's removal of bromine. In addition, the minerals in Celtic Sea Salt® aid the detoxification process. Ellen was also doing Epsom salt baths (two cups in a tub of water) twice a week and taking a magnesium supplement. "As soon as I started the salt and magnesium and the baths, I felt better. The headaches rapidly declined and my energy increased," she claimed. Three months later, Ellen's testing showed her iodide-loading test increased to

87% excretion (normal >90%) and her bromine levels fell to 35mg/24 hours. Although her bromide levels were still too high, as her iodine levels improved, her bromide levels declined. Iodine supplementation, coupled with a holistic treatment plan supporting her body's detoxification pathways enabled her to significantly improve her condition.

Ellen's case is very common. Bromide toxicity is rampant. Unless iodine levels are elevated along with the support of the body's detoxification pathways, the body will be unable to release bromide. I have seen a similar picture in numerous patients who suffer from many chronic conditions including chronic fatigue, fibromyalgia, hormone imbalances, and even cancer. These conditions significantly improve when iodine deficiency is rectified and toxic chemicals are detoxified from the body.

FLUORIDE

Fluoride, like bromide, is in the family of halogens. For over 50 years, the American Dental Association has advocated the addition of fluoride to drinking water as a preventative measure against dental caries.

However, there is much evidence to suggest that fluoride added to the water supply is ineffective at preventing caries. A study in New Zealand found that there was no difference in tooth decay rates between the fluoridated and the non-fluoridated areas.[23] This study has been repeated elsewhere. Many European countries have recognized the fallacy of adding fluoride to the water supply and have stopped the practice. The fluoridation of the water supply has been based on terrible science and is causing much more harm than good.

Fluoridation has been linked to dental fluorosis (discoloration of the teeth), hip fractures, bone cancer, lowered intelligence, kidney toxicity and other negative effects. There have been no studies that prove that long-term ingested fluoride has any positive effect.

Fluoride is known to be a toxic agent. Fluoride has been shown to inhibit the ability of the thyroid gland to concentrate iodine. [24] Fluoride was first reported to cause thyroid problems in 1854 when fluoride was found to be a cause of goiter in dogs.[25] Research has shown that fluoride is much more toxic to the body when there is iodine deficiency present.

Many commonly prescribed medications contain fluoride including the popular SSRI antidepressants such as Paxil and Prozac. Interestingly, there have been reports of this class of antidepressants increasing the risk of breast cancer.[26] Many medications that contain fluoride have been pulled from the market due to serious adverse effects. These include the cholesterol-lowering drug Baycol, Propulsid (for stomach ulcers), Posicor (anti-arrhythmic), Astemizole (allergies), Omniflox (antibiotic), Fen-Phen (weight loss) and many others. Fluoride is still used in many medications commonly prescribed including Flonase and Flovent. I believe that no medication should contain fluoride.

CHLORIDE

Chloride, like iodide, fluoride and bromide is from the family of halogens. Chloride is an important element in the extracellular fluid. There is a large amount of chloride found in the body—approximately 100gm. Chlorine (the oxidized form of chloride) is added to many products including the municipal water supply as well as to swimming pools and hot tubs as a disinfectant. It is also used as a whitener. However, chlorine is a toxic element.

A byproduct of chlorine use is the production of dioxin. Dioxin is one of the most toxic carcinogens known to mankind. It does not readily break down in the environment. Chlorine and its byproducts have been linked to birth defects, cancer[27], reproductive disorders including stillbirth,[28] and immune system breakdown.

Americans are exposed to a high level of chlorine and chlorine byproducts that are toxic to their health. This includes being exposed to the steam of the dishwasher when the door is opened after cleaning (chlorine superheated and combined with detergent). In addition, the sugar-substitute Sucralose (Splenda®) contains chlorinated table sugar.

No one denies the importance of having clean drinking and swimming pool water that is free of bacteria. However, there are many safer alternatives to disinfecting water including the use of iodine, hydrogen peroxide, ultraviolet light, and ozone that could be substituted for chlorine.

PERCHLORATE

Perchlorate consists of one atom of chlorine surrounded by four atoms of oxygen. It is found naturally in the environment and can be man-made. Perchlorate can displace iodine binding in the body. It can damage the iodine transport mechanism (NIS).[29] Perchlorate, at low levels, has been found to cause thyroid cancer, goiter, hypothyroidism, and disruption of the normal menstrual cycle, as well as a weakening of the immune system.[30]

Perchlorate is used in a variety of products including car air bags, leather tanning, and fireworks. Today, one of the main manufacturing uses of perchlorate is for rocket fuel.

Sixty years ago, perchlorate was used as a medical treatment for hyperthyroidism. In large enough doses, the chlorine in perchlorate will displace iodine. Without iodine, the thyroid gland will become inactive. In the 1960's, due to safety concerns, perchlorate use in medicine was discontinued.

Perchlorate exposure has been associated with many serious health conditions (see below). These conditions all relate to lowered iodine levels when there is excess perchlorate in the body.

Some Consequences of Perchlorate
Breast disease
Hypothyroidism
Immune System Problems
Mental retardation in newborns
Poor fetal development
Poor neonatal development
Thyroid cancer

Today, perchlorate still continues to cause significant health problems. Ground water is contaminated throughout much of the United States from manufactured perchlorate. Ninety percent of the perchlorate manufactured each year is used for rocket fuel for NASA, defense contractors and the Air Force.[31] Most perchlorate has been disposed directly into the ground or into abandoned mines.[32] [33]

The entire lower Colorado River is contaminated with perchlorate. The lower Colorado River irrigates more than 1.8 million acres of land which encompasses over 15% of the nation's crops and 13% of the nation's livestock. Approximately 20 million Americans drink water from the Colorado River which is contaminated with perchlorate. In fact, at least 43 states have contaminated water from perchlorate.[34] When perchlorate is released into the water supply, it can persist for long periods of time.

Researchers compared thyroid function in newborns that live in an area (Yuma, Arizona) with perchlorate-contaminated drinking water supplied from the lower Colorado River versus newborns from an area (Flagstaff, Arizona) with non-contaminated drinking water. Rocket and missile facilities were thought to be the source of perchlorate that contaminated the water. Fifteen hundred infants were studied. The results showed that infants in Yuma were found to have significantly depressed thyroid function as compared to infants from Flagstaff.[35] Perchlorate levels were found to be elevated (above EPA limits) in the water supply in Yuma and undetectable in the water supply in Flagstaff.[36] Perchlorate is known to cross the placenta and can cause in-utero thyroid abnormalities.[37] Thyroid abnormalities in utero or at birth are the leading cause of preventable mental retardation.[38]

Drinking water is not the only problem with perchlorate. Lettuce grown in the fall and winter months in the southwestern United States contains very high amounts of perchlorate. Up to 70% of the nation's fall and winter lettuce supply is irrigated with perchlorate-contaminated water from the lower Colorado River.

Over 130 samples of commercial lettuce were tested for perchlorate. This included head lettuce as well as adult and baby greens grown both organically and conventionally. Significant amounts of perchlorate were found in 83% of the lettuce samples tested. There was virtually no difference between organically or conventionally grown lettuce. It is estimated that by eating lettuce during the winter months, 1.6 million American women of childbearing age are exposed to more perchlorate than the EPA's recommended safe dose.[39]

Perchlorate has also been found in dairy and human milk. Forty seven dairy milk samples from 11 states were examined for perchlorate. Significant amounts of perchlorate were found in 98% of the samples (46/47). Thirty six human milk samples from 18 states were examined for perchlorate. All of the human milk samples -100%- were found to contain measurable amounts of perchlorate. The mean perchlorate level of human milk was 500% higher than dairy milk. In fact, there was an inverse correlation of perchlorate and iodide in breast milk; the higher the perchlorate level, the lower the iodide level. Breast milk is the only source of iodide in a breast-fed infant. The high perchlorate levels found in this study prompted the authors to conclude, "Recommended iodine intake by pregnant and lactating women may need to be revised upward."[40]

As mentioned in Chapter 2, iodine levels have fallen over 50% in the United States over the last 30 years. There is no doubt that part of this decline can be attributed to increasing exposure to toxic goitrogens such as perchlorate.

HOW TO DETOXIFY PERCHLORATE

Perchlorate is a chlorine-containing substance. Chlorine is part of the family of halides—iodine, bromine, and chlorine. Iodine levels can competitively inhibit perchlorate and result in perchlorate being excreted from the body. Ensuring an adequate intake of iodine and iodine sufficiency for the body is the best protection against any toxic halide, including perchlorate. Furthermore, ingesting adequate amounts of vitamins, minerals and Vitamin C can help any detoxification program.

PUTTING IT ALL TOGETHER: STUDYING THE IODINE STATUS AND HALOGEN STATUS IN EIGHT PATIENTS

Iodine is not only deficient in our diets, it is being crowded out by the other halogens mentioned above: bromine, fluoride and perchlorate. These toxic halogens are making a bad situation (iodine deficiency) worse. How toxic are our bodies from these halogens?

I undertook a study to look at the level of halides, iodide, fluoride, and bromide in eight patients. My theory was that most individuals are lacking in iodine and are toxic from the other halogens (bromide and fluoride). The patients were selected at random from my practice.

None of these patients had been treated with iodine before this study. It is known that iodine can compete with the other halogens for binding in the body. Therefore, if there is a sufficient amount of iodine present, then the toxic halogens (i.e., bromide, fluoride) should not be able to bind in the body, and they will be excreted. The patients were studied at baseline to look not only at their iodine levels but also at their bromide and fluoride levels. After taking a loading dose of iodine (50mg of iodide/iodine),

116

they were rechecked for their levels of iodine, bromide and fluoride. Next, the patients took a daily dose of iodine (50mg of iodine/iodide in the form of Iodoral®) for 30 days and they repeated a 24-hour urine collection. The results are summarized below. As can be seen from the table below, little iodine was excreted at baseline. The data indicated that all of these patients were iodine deficient at baseline.

Average Measurement of Urinary Excretion of Halides with Iodine Supplementation in Eight Patients

	Baseline	1 Day	30 Days
Fluoride mg/24 hours	1.07	1.91	1.95
Bromide mg/24 hours	17.06	25.44	26.63
Iodide mg/24 hours	0.08	20.13	33.05
% Iodine excretion	N/A	40.2%	66.1%

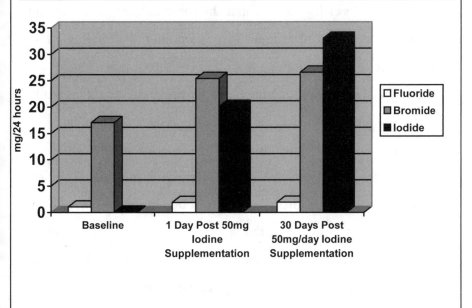

After ingesting 50 mg/day of an iodide/iodine supplement (Iodoral®), repeat testing was done on day 1 and after 30 days of supplementation. As expected, as iodine was supplemented, the excretion of iodine increased—from 40.2% to 66.1%. Increasing the iodine load increased the excretion of bromide and fluoride. This shows that the body was adapting to the iodine load and becoming saturated with iodine while at the same time detoxifying from the toxic halides, bromide and fluoride.

In an iodine sufficient state, normally 90% (45mg) of the loading dose of iodine ingested will be excreted, while 10% (5mg) will be retained. Although an iodine-sufficient state was not reached with these patients, their levels at 30 days showed an improved excretion rate. My experience has shown that in an iodine deficient state, it takes from three to six months of iodine supplementation before iodine saturation is reached.

It is interesting to note that the toxic halides, bromide and fluoride, were excreted at much larger amounts than iodide. The baseline level of bromide was nearly three times the ADI (Average Daily Intake) recommended by researchers.[41] This study shows how prevalent these toxic items are in our environment.

The data also shows that after one day of supplementation, bromide excretion increased nearly 50% and fluoride excretion increased 78%, while the average excretion of iodide was 40%, which is very low. This would indicate that iodine supplementation has a detoxifying effect on the body. This detoxifying effect helps the body release toxic items such as fluoride and bromide. After one month of supplementation, iodine excretion improved to 66% (normal excretion of iodine is >90%).

The most important facet of iodine supplementation is that it helps patients improve their health and helps them feel better. This is due to the positive effects iodine has on the thyroid and the immune system, as well as the detoxifying effects iodine has on toxic items such as bromide and fluoride. In many patients, I have also observed the detoxifying effect of iodine supplementation on mercury and other heavy metals.

ARE THE TOXIC HALOGENS FLUORIDE AND BROMINE RESPONSIBLE FOR THE EPIDEMIC RISE IN BREAST CANCER?

The research is clear that bromine and fluoride are toxic items for the body. In an iodine deficient state, the toxicity of bromide and fluoride are exacerbated.

I undertook a study in my office to look at the difference in iodide, bromine and fluoride levels in eight women with breast cancer versus ten women without breast cancer. Urinary levels of bromine and fluoride were measured at baseline, one day after taking 50mg of iodine/iodide (Iodoral®) and 30 days after taking 50mg/day of iodine/iodide (Iodoral®). The results shocked me.

Iodine levels were low in all of the women tested. This is not surprising because, as previously described in this book, the rates of iodine deficiency are at epidemic proportions.

What shocked me was the difference in the levels of the toxic halogens bromide and fluoride. Bromide levels were found to be significantly elevated in the breast cancer versus the non-breast cancer subjects. The table and graph below show the bromide results.

Bromide Excretion in 8 Breast Cancer and 10 Non-Breast Cancer Subjects

	Baseline	1 Day Post 50mg I	30 Days Post 50mg/day I
Bromide (mg/24 hours) Breast Cancer	18.81	26.25	26.73
Bromide (mg/24 hours) Non-Breast Cancer	11.3	15.82	16.7

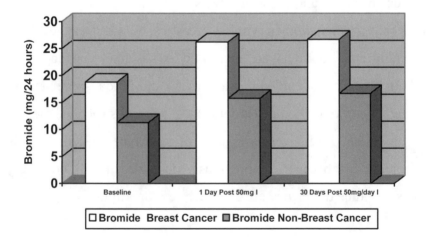

The fluoride results (next page) showed similar results, with the breast cancer subjects exhibiting higher fluoride levels as compared to the non-breast cancer subjects. Although the difference in the fluoride levels were not as dramatic as the bromide levels, this data shows that breast cancer patients are absorbing and retaining larger amounts of toxic halides as compared to non-breast cancer subjects.

Fluoride Excretion in 8 Breast Cancer and 10 Non-Breast Cancer Subjects

Fluoride (mg/24 hours) Breast Cancer	1.49	1.84	1.10
Fluoride (mg/24 hours) Non Breast Cancer	1.13	1.24	1.30

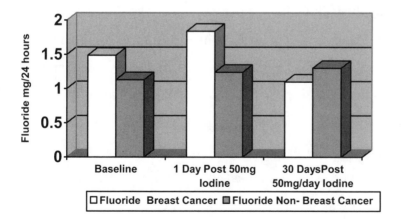

The way to reduce the body's burden of toxic halides is to increase the body's iodine levels. As previously mentioned, the toxicity of fluoride and bromine will be exacerbated in an iodine-deficient state.

The use of iodine supplementation, along with a holistic nutritional program which facilitates the detoxification abilities of the body will allow the body to decrease its levels of toxic halides.

FINAL THOUGHTS

We are in the midst of a cancer epidemic. At the present time, one in three Americans will get cancer. Cancer is not caused by chemotherapy, radiation and surgery deficiency. Cancer is a multifactorial illness that will only be conquered when the underlying causes of cancer are properly thought out and thoroughly dealt with.

There is no doubt that our exposure to toxic chemicals is increasing at the same time our nutrient status is declining. Is it any wonder that cancer rates are reaching epidemic proportions? Currently one in seven women (14%) has breast cancer and one in three men (33%) has prostate cancer. Iodine deficiency coupled with the increasing toxic load in our bodies could explain a great deal about why these cancer numbers are so high.

Iodine supplementation has multiple positive effects on the body. These positive effects are found in many different illnesses from fatigue states to autoimmune disorders and cancer. It is important not only to ensure adequate levels of nutrients in the body, but also to help the body utilize these nutrients by enhancing the detoxification mechanisms. Iodine supplementation will not only provide a valuable nutrient for the body it will also aid in the detoxification process of the body.

[1] Levin, M. Bromide psychosis: four varieties. Am. J. Psych. 104:798-804, 1948

[2] Clark. G. Applied Pharmacology. Churchill, London. 1938

[3] Sangster, B., et al. The influence of sodium bromide in man: A study in human volunteers with special emphasis on the endocrine and the central nervous system. Fd. Chem. Toxic., 21: 409-419, 1983

[4] Van Leeuwen, FX. The toxicology of bromide ion. Crit. Rev. Toxicol. 1987;18:189-213

[5] CAS Registry number: 74:83:9

[6] Horowitz, B. Bromism from excessive cola consumption. Clinical Toxicology, 35 (3), 315-320. 1997

[7] Pavelka, S. High bromide intake affects the accumulation of iodide in the rat thyroid and skin. Biol. Trace elem. Res. 2001. summer;82(1-3):133

[8] Pavalka, S. Effect of high bromide levels in the organism on the biological half-life of iodine in the rat. Biol. Trace elem. Res. 2001. summer;82(1-3):133

[9] Buchberger, W. Effects of sodium bromide on the biosynthesis of thyroid hormones and brominated/iodinated thyronines. J. Trace Elem. Elec. Health Dis. Vol.4. 1990, p. 25-30

[10] London, W.T. Bread- a dietary source of large quantities of iodine. New. Engl. J. Med. 273:381, 1965

[11] Abraham, G. The effect of ingestion of inorganic nonradioactive iodine/iodide in patients with simple goiter and in Graves' disease: A review of published studies compared with current trends. Optimox Research. 9.09.03

[12] Vobecky, M. Effect of enhanced bromide intake on the-concentration ratio I/Br in the rat thyroid gland. Bio. Trace Element Research, 43:509-513, 1994

[13] Abraham, G. IBID. 9.09.03

[14] CDC. National Center for Health Statistics. Cdc.gov

[15] Hollowell, Je. Iodine nutrition in the United States. Trends and public health implications: Iodine excretion data from National Health and Nutrition Examination surveys I and III. J. Clin. Endocrinol. Metab. 83:3401-3408, 1998

[16] vobecky, M. Effect of enhanced bromide intake on the concentration ratio I/Br in the rat thyroid gland. Bo. Trace. Element Res.: 1994

[17] Abraham, G. Iodine supplementation markedly increases urinary excretion of fluoride and bromide. Letter to the editor. Townsend Letter for Doctors and Patients. May 2003

[18] Abraham, G. IBID. 2003

[19] Rauws, AG. Pharmacokinetics of bromine ion—an overview. Fd Chem. Toxic. 1983;21:379-382

[20] Sticht, G. Bromine. In: Handbook on toxicity of inorganic compounds. Seiler, Hg, et al, editors. Marcel Dekker Inc. 1988;143-151

[21] Sensenbach, W. J. Am. Med. Assoc. Vol. 125. 1944. 769-772

[22] Rauws, A.G. Pharmacokinetics of bromine ion-an overview. Chem. Toxic. Vol. 21, No. 1. 379. 1983

[23] Colquhoun, G. New Evidence on fluoridation. Social Science and Medicine. 19. 1239-46. 1984.

[24] Galletti, P. Effect of fluorine on thyroidal iodine metabolism in hyperthyroidism

[25] Maumene, e. Experience pour determiner l'action des fluores sur l'econimie animale. Compt. Rend. Acad. Sci (Paris) 39:538-539. 1854

[26] 35th Annual Meeting of the Society for Epidemiologic Research, Seattle, WA. June 2000.

[27] Epidemiology. 1998;9(1): 21-28, 29-35.

[28] Epidemiology. May 1999. 10:233-237

[29] Tonacchera, M. Relative potencies and additivity of perchlorate, thiocyanate, nitrate and iodide on the inhibition of radioactive iodide uptake by the human sodium iodide symporter. Thyroid. 2004. 14. 1012-19

[30] EPA. Perchlorate environmental contamination: toxicological review and risk characterization based on emerging information. 1998

[31] EPA. 1998. IBID.

[32] Journal of the Am. Water Works Ass. 1957. 49(10):1334-1342

[33] Environmental Working Group, 2005. From www.ewg.com.

[34] Environmental Working Group, 2005. From www.ewg.com.

[35] Ross, B. Ammonium perchlorate contamination of Colorado River drinking water is associated with abnormal thyroid function in newborns in Arizona. J. of Occup. And Env. Medicine. Vol 42(8). August, 2000. p. 777-782

[36] U.S. EPA. Regional Agency 9 Lab. USEPA;August 16, 1999

[37] Fisher, D. Maternal-fetal thyroid function in pregnancy. Clin. Perinat. 1983;10:615026

[38] WHO.

[39] Envirnonmental Working Group. IBID. 2005.

[40] Kirk, Andrea. Perchlorate and iodide in dairy and breast milk. Environ. Sci and Technol. 2000.

[41] Van Leeuwen, F., et al. The effect of sodium bromide on thyroid function. Arch. Toxic. Suppl. 12:93-97. 1988

Chapter 6

*Iodine and the
Thyroid Gland*

CHAPTER 6: IODINE AND THE THYROID GLAND

Iodine is an essential ingredient in all of the thyroid hormones. T4 (thyroxine) contains four iodine molecules. T3 (triiodothyronine) contains three iodine molecules. Without sufficient iodine supply, the thyroid gland is unable to make thyroid hormones in adequate amounts.

The thyroid gland cannot optimally function in an iodine-deficient state. One of the consequences of an iodine-deficient state is goiter (swelling of the thyroid gland). Over a hundred years ago, it was shown that goiter could be avoided and often reversed by giving iodine. In addition to goiter formation, iodine deficiency may also lead to hypothyroidism and autoimmune thyroid diseases including Graves' and Hashimoto's disease. Studies have shown that iodine-deficient individuals have an increased incidence of antithyroid antibodies.[1][2]

Iodine is found in minute quantities in the body, with approximately 15-20mg in the thyroid of the average adult, when iodine levels are sufficient.[3][4] Due to its dependence on iodine to make thyroid hormone, the thyroid gland has developed a specialized system to concentrate iodine, and it is able to concentrate a large amount of iodine as compared to its size. This system is known as the sodium/iodide symporter. The breasts also use this same mechanism to concentrate iodine.

The thyroid gland is regulated by the pituitary gland. The pituitary gland releases a hormone, thyroid stimulating hormone (TSH). TSH stimulates the thyroid gland to release thyroxine (T4). Triiodothyronine (T3) is converted from T4 in the periphery of the body. T3 is believed to be the active form of thyroid hormone that drives the metabolic functions of thyroid hormone. The Figure below illustrates this process.

Pituitary gland ⟶ TSH ⟶ Thyroid Gland ⟶ T4 ⟶ T3

T4 and T3 are the thyroid hormones. The '4' in T4 and the '3' in T3 refer to the number of iodine molecules present. As previously stated, T4 has four iodine molecules present, while T3

130

has three iodine molecules present. Without adequate iodine levels, the thyroid gland is unable to produce adequate thyroid hormone. The end result of an iodine deficiency can be a poorly functioning thyroid gland, goiter, increased autoimmune thyroid problems, and an increased risk of thyroid cancer.

Thyroid hormone is essential for normal brain development of the newborn. Since iodine is necessary for the production of thyroid hormone, an iodine-deficient state may predispose the newborn to abnormal brain development. In children, iodine deficiency can result in mental retardation as well as goiter. Research has found almost a 50% increase in perinatal mortality due to iodine deficiency.[5]

Many studies have shown that children who live in iodine-deficient areas have lower IQ's as compared to children living in iodine sufficient areas. A large analysis comparing children in iodine deficient and iodine sufficient areas showed a 13.5 point difference in IQ score.[6]

Iodine is also necessary for the proper function of the adult thyroid gland. It is impossible for the thyroid gland to function optimally in an iodine-deficient state.

Janet, age 57, had been treated for hypothyroidism for two years. She was recently found to be deficient in iodine and given a therapeutic trial of a combination of iodine and iodide (Iodoral®). I asked her to write to me a letter about her experience with iodine. She wrote me the following letter.

"After taking Armour thyroid for over two years, I began to feel somewhat sluggish and felt that perhaps I needed more thyroid hormone. Dr. Brownstein told me to take two tablets of iodine (the tablets were a mixture of iodine and iodide) with my thyroid medicine. It has been over five months since I began the iodine treatment and I still feel the perkiness everyday that I have been looking for. In fact, I started to feel better the first day that I took the iodine. The iodine certainly was needed. I am just thrilled about how much better I feel."

WHAT ABOUT IODIZED SALT?

As mentioned in Chapter 2, iodine was added to iodized salt over 70 years ago to combat goiter and cretinism. The RDA to combat these illnesses was established at (150ug/day) with one goal in mind: prevent goiter and cretinism. The RDA for iodine has been successful at combating goiter and cretinism; however, the RDA is woefully inadequate in preventing many other thyroid disorders including hypothyroidism, as well as Graves' and Hashimoto's disease. Other illnesses associated with iodine deficiency (e.g., breast cancer, fibrocystic breast disease) are covered in other chapters.

HOW COMMON ARE THYROID PROBLEMS?

Thyroid illnesses are found at ever increasing numbers. Recent studies have estimated that 10% of the adult population of the United States (13 million) may have laboratory evidence of thyroid disease.[7] I have written in my book, ***Overcoming Thyroid Disorders,*** that I believe these numbers are too low and probably approach 30-40% (up to 52 million adult Americans).[8]

Why is adequate thyroid hormone so important? Every single cell, muscle, and organ in the body depends on adequate thyroid hormone levels for optimal functioning. Thyroid hormone acts as the body's major metabolic regulator. In a low thyroid state, known as hypothyroidism, the thyroid gland is releasing inadequate amounts of thyroid hormone to meet the body's metabolic demands, and the metabolic rate is therefore reduced. In a hyperthyroid state, the thyroid gland is releasing excess amounts of thyroid hormone that results in an elevated metabolic rate.

How could so many people across this country and the world have a serious problem like a thyroid disorder? Although the etiology of thyroid illness can be varied, one common denominator may be iodine deficiency.

As previously discussed in Chapter 2, one-third of the world's population lives in an iodine deficient area by World Health Organization (WHO) standards. This number of people living in an iodine deficient area closely correlates with the estimates for the number of people who have thyroid disorders. All individuals with a thyroid disorder should be screened for iodine deficiency.

HYPOTHYROIDISM

The thyroid gland controls the metabolic activity of the

body. When there is adequate thyroid hormone available for the cells of the body, there is a normal metabolic activity present. By contrast, in a hypothyroid state, there is a lowered metabolic activity present. The table below lists some of the signs and symptoms of hypothyroidism.

As previously mentioned, the main thyroid hormones T4 and T3 each require iodine's presence to be produced. In an iodine deficient state, hypothyroidism is much more common. My research has shown that iodine levels need to be investigated in all hypothyroid individuals. If iodine is found to be deficient, many times reversing the iodine deficient condition can result in improving or even curing the hypothyroid condition.

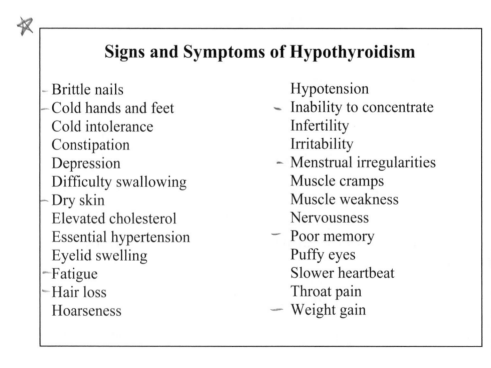

Signs and Symptoms of Hypothyroidism

Brittle nails	Hypotension
Cold hands and feet	Inability to concentrate
Cold intolerance	Infertility
Constipation	Irritability
Depression	Menstrual irregularities
Difficulty swallowing	Muscle cramps
Dry skin	Muscle weakness
Elevated cholesterol	Nervousness
Essential hypertension	Poor memory
Eyelid swelling	Puffy eyes
Fatigue	Slower heartbeat
Hair loss	Throat pain
Hoarseness	Weight gain

Iodine and thyroid hormone have a synergistic action in the hypothyroid patient. When it is indicated, it is more effective to use iodine along with thyroid hormone to achieve the best results.

Karen, age 50, suffered with hypothyroidism for 15 years. Her symptoms included fatigue, mental confusion, puffiness, and hair loss. I diagnosed Karen with hypothyroidism three years ago and began treating her with Armour thyroid and a combination of vitamins, minerals, and herbs. She noticed a significant improvement in her symptoms when she began taking Armour thyroid. "I feel like I got my life back. I could think much more clearly and my energy level started to improve," she said. Karen's daughter, Lisa (22 years old) had similar symptoms and was diagnosed with hypothyroidism two years ago. She had similar positive results with thyroid supplementation. Four months ago, the laboratory tests showed both Karen and Lisa had iodine deficiency. Three months after starting iodine supplementation, I received a letter from Karen that said in part, "Lisa and I take Armour thyroid and we have had much success with that, but adding iodine really made a difference. We have more energy and it is much easier to get up in the morning. The muscle stiffness I occasionally experienced is gone. As you know, I spent three weeks in California with my mom who had undergone surgery for colon cancer. I was in a bed other than my own and I was on a different time schedule. I wasn't getting much sleep and the stress level was very high. In the past, a situation like that would have exhausted my body and I would be aching all the time. Not this time! In spite of everything that was going on, I felt great. I attribute that to the iodine, because it is the only change I have made since being in California. Lisa's experience has been similar. She is in college and has a very irregular schedule. Since she started taking iodine, I have a noticed a big difference in her energy level. She actually wakes up on her own and has much more energy during the day and night." After two months of therapy, I had asked Karen and Lisa to reduce their iodine dosage slightly and they did not feel as good. *"When Lisa and I cut down our dosage of iodine, we gradually noticed we did not feel as well. At your recommendation, we increased the dosage and began to feel as good as we were before,"* Karen wrote. Karen and Lisa's experience is very common for many of my other patients. As is the case with Karen and Lisa, proper iodine levels are necessary in order to have optimal thyroid function.

GRAVES' AND HASHIMOTO'S DISEASE

Graves' disease is an autoimmune illness whereby the thyroid gland is attacked by the body's antibodies. This causes an inflammation and swelling of the thyroid gland. Hyperthyroidism, (an overactive metabolic state) is common in Graves' disease.

Graves' disease occurs in 0.25-1% of the population and the number of individuals diagnosed with Graves' disease is increasing. Graves' is more common in females and usually occurs in middle age. In conventional medicine, there is no known cause of Graves' disease. Some causative factors reported in the literature include a genetic predisposition, infections, and stress.

Hashimoto's disease is also an autoimmune illness where the body produces antithyroid peroxidase antibodies (anti-TPO) that cause an inflammation of the thyroid gland. The end result is goiter formation in many, and hypothyroidism is usually the end result of long-standing Hashimoto's disease.

Hashimoto's disease is more prevalent than Graves' disease, occurring in 0.1-5% of the population. The incidence of Hashimoto's disease is rising rapidly. In conventional medicine, there is no known cause of Hashimoto's disease, and the causative factors are similar to those reported above for Graves' disease.

The rising incidence of Hashimoto's and Graves' disease correlates with falling iodine levels. I believe the increase in both Hashimoto's and Graves' disease, occurring at near epidemic rates, is because of iodine deficiency.

Researchers in Europe reported on the incidence of hyperthyroidism in two areas of Denmark (Aalborg and Copenhagen). The two areas were chosen because Aalborg had slightly lower iodine levels (53μg/L—measured on urinary excretion) as compared to Copenhagen (68μg/L). The results are summarized on the next page.

Iodine Excretion in Two Areas of Denmark

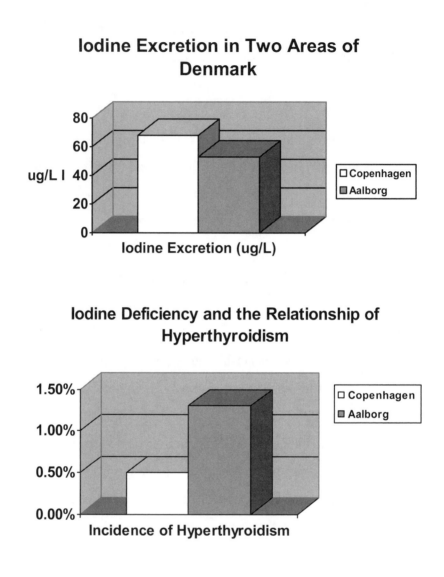

ug/L I

80
60
40
20
0

Iodine Excretion (ug/L)

□ Copenhagen
■ Aalborg

Iodine Deficiency and the Relationship of Hyperthyroidism

1.50%
1.00%
0.50%
0.00%

Incidence of Hyperthyroidism

□ Copenhagen
■ Aalborg

For comparison to the Denmark results, the average iodide excretion in the U.S. is 145µg/L with over 12% of the U.S. population below 50 µg/L. In the U.S., 16.5% of women in their reproductive age have a markedly low iodide excretion below 50μg/L[9]. The World Health Organization (WHO) claims iodide excretion below 50μg/L is classified as moderate/severe iodide deficiency.[10]

If iodine caused autoimmune thyroid problems, you would expect the rate of hyperthyroidism to decline as iodine levels fall. That is just not the case. This study clearly shows that lowered iodine levels in Aalborg are associated with a 260% elevated incidence of autoimmune thyroid problems (hyperthyroidism) when compared to an area with slightly higher iodine levels-- Copenhagen.[11]

CONVENTIONAL APPROACHES TO AUTOIMMUNE THYROID DISEASE: RADIOACTIVE IODINE

The conventional approach to treating autoimmune thyroid disorders revolves primarily around alleviating the symptoms of the autoimmune illness, mainly the symptoms of hyperthyroidism. This includes the use of antithyroid drugs (e.g., Propylthiouracil, Methimazole) that block the production of thyroid hormone. Other conventional treatments include surgery and radioactive iodine. Both of these modalities work by reducing the volume of thyroid tissue. However, neither of these treatments addresses the underlying causative factor(s) of these illnesses. In fact, in conventional medicine, there is rarely a search for an underlying causative factor(s). If you don't search for an underlying causative factor, then how can you formulate an effective treatment plan?

Radioactive iodine is the preferred method in conventional medicine for treating autoimmune thyroid disorders.[12] In one of the most respected books on thyroid problems, radioactive iodine is reported as "effective, safe, and relatively inexpensive"[13]. Let's look at all three of these claims.

IS RADIOACTIVE IODINE EFFECTIVE?

If the goal of treating an autoimmune thyroid disorder is to destroy the thyroid gland, then yes, radioactive iodine is effective. It is well known that iodine is taken up by the thyroid gland. By using a radioactive form of iodine (I^{131}), the theory is that wherever the radioactive form of iodine binds, the radioactivity will destroy the surrounding cells. In the case of autoimmune thyroid disorders, the binding of the radioactive iodine to the thyroid gland will result in the destruction of thyroid tissue by the radioactive isotope.

If the cause of autoimmune thyroid disorders is too much thyroid tissue that needs to be destroyed, then the use of radioactive iodine could be considered effective. However, excess thyroid tissue is not the cause of autoimmune thyroid disorders; it is a consequence of the illness.

Radioactive iodine has never been considered a treatment to change the underlying cause of the illness. Radioactive iodine is solely a palliative treatment for the hyperthyroid symptoms of autoimmune thyroid problems. I believe there are more effective ways to treat autoimmune thyroid illnesses using natural items, which will be covered below.

IS RADIOACTIVE IODINE SAFE?

Not only will radioactive iodine bind to the thyroid gland destroying thyroid cells, it will also bind to other sites in the body besides the thyroid gland. It was established in Chapter 1 that iodine is present in all of the cells of the body. Radioactive iodine will be concentrated where iodine is concentrated in the body, including the breasts in women. With breast cancer at epidemic rates (1/7 women), I believe no therapy should be used that may potentially increase this rate. There are safer alternatives.

RADIOACTIVE IODINE: IS IT INEXPENSIVE?

The cost of radioactive iodine is approximately $3,000. Radioactive iodine is an expensive procedure that does not address the underlying cause of the illness. There are much better alternatives than radioactive iodine.

SEARCHING FOR AN UNDERLYING CAUSE OF AUTOIMMUNE THYROID PROBLEMS

In order to formulate an effective, safe, and inexpensive treatment for autoimmune thyroid problems, one must first search for an underlying cause of the illness. As I discussed in my book,

Overcoming Thyroid Disorders, the underlying cause(s) of autoimmune thyroid disorders can be varied. This can include infections, toxicities, food allergies (i.e., gluten intolerance), and nutritional imbalances. I believe that iodine deficiency may be an important factor in developing an autoimmune thyroid problem.

Tracy, 40-years-old, was diagnosed with Hashimoto's disease ten years ago after the birth of her son. Her TSH elevated to 150mU/l (normal 0.2-4.7mU/l) and she felt miserable. "I could not think clearly. I felt like my brain was in a fog. I would go to the store and not know why I was there. I was also extremely fatigued", she said. She had symptoms of hyperthyroid and hypothyroid problems. "Sometimes my heart would start racing for no apparent reason. I was irritable and moody. I couldn't work out because I felt so poorly," she claimed. Tracy was placed on Synthroid, but felt no better. Although her laboratory tests improved and her TSH became normal, none of her symptoms improved. When I began treating Tracy, I found an allergy to gluten. I placed her on a gluten-free diet that alleviated many of her symptoms. She was also given nutritional supplements to correct many vitamin and mineral imbalances. Tracy's thyroid medication was changed to a more natural thyroid prescription and she improved. "I felt much better. I could think more clearly. Most importantly, my energy came back," she said. When I investigated her iodine status, Tracy was found to be markedly iodine deficient. With the use of a combination of iodine/iodide, she further improved. Tracy claimed, "When I started taking iodine, my energy improved. I was sleeping better and dreaming better. I started to lift weights and build muscle which I haven't been able to do in a long time. I cannot believe the positive changes that I have seen with the iodine." Tracy's iodine levels have improved with using a combination of iodine/iodide and she continues to supplement today.

Marlene, a 45-year-old advertising executive, was diagnosed with Graves' disease one year ago. "I woke up one morning and my heart was beating very fast and I felt like I was on too much caffeine," she said. Marlene went to her physician who diagnosed her with Graves' disease. "I asked him what caused it, and he couldn't answer me. When he told me he wanted to treat me with radioactive iodine, I questioned him. I wasn't satisfied with his answers and I began to look at the alternatives," she said. Marlene was diagnosed with iodine deficiency (24% excretion on an Iodine loading test—normal levels >90%). She was also found to have multiple nutritional deficiencies and mercury toxicity. I treated Marlene with iodine (Iodoral®) and vitamins and minerals. In addition, a mercury detoxification plan was implemented. Marlene also improved her diet, eliminating refined carbohydrates and drinking more water. After four weeks on this therapy, she noticed a dramatic improvement in her symptoms. "I was thrilled. All of the hyper symptoms resolved. I began to feel much better and even my energy level went up. People began asking me what I was doing, since they thought I looked so much *better," she said. Marlene's case is not unique. Graves' disease can be treated effectively with a comprehensive holistic program.*

My initial study on the iodine status of 24 patients (see Chapter 2) showed that 92% of those with Hashimoto's and Graves' disease also had iodine deficiency. Nearly every one of these patients had dramatic improvements in their symptoms with the use of a combination of iodine/iodide to replace the body's deficit. Rarely do I see a negative side effect from the replacement of a natural form of iodine, and side effects are easily rectified with adjusting the dosage.

Inorganic, non-radioactive iodine (such as Lugol's or Iodoral®) has been used to treat autoimmune thyroid problems for over 100 years. There are numerous reports in the literature citing the beneficial effects of iodine. In fact, iodine has been shown to reduce the hyperplasia and hypervascularity characteristic of Graves' disease.[14] In cases of hyperthyroidism, milligram doses of iodine/iodide were used effectively prior to thyroid surgery to decrease thyroid hormone blood levels and prevent thyroid storm.

There is a concern that the use of iodine in an autoimmune thyroid patient can exacerbate the symptoms of thyroid toxicosis. However, with proper dosing and close monitoring, this side effect is very rare. Negative effects from iodine can usually be resolved by adjusting the dosage.

FINAL THOUGHTS

I believe all individuals with a thyroid problem should have their iodine levels checked. If iodine levels are suboptimal, iodine replacement with the correct form of iodine should be instituted. My experience has clearly shown that the appropriate use of iodine in treating thyroid disorders, from hypothyroidism to Graves' and Hashimoto's disease, is not only safe, but effective and inexpensive. This is a holistic way to search for and treat an underlying cause of thyroid problems with a safe and natural agent. But, most importantly, people improve their condition without experiencing any serious adverse effects.

Clinical experience has shown that when iodine is added to a hypothyroid patient's regimen, it may become necessary to adjust their thyroid dosage. Approximately one-third of patients being treated for hypothyroidism will need to lower their dose of thyroid hormone when an iodine deficient disorder is corrected. The other two-thirds of people taking thyroid hormone can usually maintain their dosage of thyroid hormone. Also, patients with Graves' and Hashimoto's disease may have to adjust their thyroid medications.

Iodine replacement is not the only therapy for thyroid illness. Nutritional supplementation, detoxification, drinking adequate amounts of water and diet changes can also help these conditions. I refer the reader to my book, ***Overcoming Thyroid Disorders*** for more information.

[1] Fenzi, F. Role of autoimmune and familial factors in goiter prevalence. Studies performed in moderately endemic area. J. Endocrin. Invest. 9:131-164. 1986

[2] Eur. J. Endocr. 2000 Oct; 143(4):485-991

[3] Delange, F. Werner and Ingbar's The Thyroid. Lippincott Williams and Wilkins. 2000.

[4] Herzel, B. Modern Nutrition in Health and Disease. 1998

[5] Thilly, C.G. Bull. Acad. Med. Belg. 1981;136:389

[6] Herzel, B. Modern Nutrition in Health and Disease. 1998

[7] Canaris, Gay, et al. The Colorado Thyroid Disease Prevalence Study. Arch. Intern. Med. Vol 160, Feb 28, 2000

[8] Brownstein, D. Overcoming Thyroid Disorders. Medical Alt. Press. 2002

[9] Hollowell et al., J Clin Endocrinol Metab 83:3401-3408, 1998

[10] WHO. Assessment of iodine deficiency disorders and monitoring their elimination, 2nd Edition. 2001.

[11] Eur. J. Endocr. 2000. Oct;143(4):485-91

[12] Solomon, B. Current trends in the management of Graves' disease. J. Clin. Endocrn. Metab. 1990:70:1518

[13] Cooper, D. In Werner and Ingbar's The Thyroid. 2000. Lippincott, Williams and Wilkins.

[14] Aceves, C. Is iodine a gatekeeper of the integrity of the mammary gland? J. of mammary gland biol. and neoplasia. Vol. 10, No2. April 2005

Chapter 7

Iodine Dosage Guidelines

CHAPTER 7: IODINE DOSAGE GUIDELINES

Now that we have established that the RDA for iodine (approximately 150ug/day) is inadequate, how much iodine should you take? There is some concern in the conventional literature that too much iodine can harm the thyroid gland and cause other problems in the body. This chapter will explore how to safely use iodine to achieve your optimal health.

The question of dosage cannot be answered without reviewing the iodine intake of the Japanese (covered in more detail in Chapter 4). It has been estimated that the mainland Japanese ingest approximately 13.8mg of iodine per day, which is approximately 100 times the RDA.[1] The Japanese receive most of their iodine from seaweed, which is known to concentrate iodine.

What is the effect of ingesting this larger amount of iodine? The Japanese who consume these large amounts (by U.S. RDA standards) of iodine have remarkably lower levels of breast, endometrial, and ovarian cancers. In addition, there is a significantly lower amount of fibrocystic breast disease in Japanese women who consume the larger amount of iodine. Mainland Japanese men have a significantly lower rate of prostate cancer as compared to the U.S. male population including Japanese males who have migrated to the United States. The medical literature has pointed out a possible relationship between all of these cancers and iodine deficiency.

CONCERN WITH USING HIGH LEVELS OF IODINE

There is some concern that the ingestion of iodine in excess of the RDA (approximately 150ug/day) will cause adverse effects. I will show you that with the proper monitoring and dosing of iodine, it is safe and effective to use at doses above the RDA. There are seven major concerns with using iodine in excess of the RDA:

1. Allergy
2. Autoimmune thyroid disease
3. Detoxification reactions
4. Iodine-induced hypothyroidism and goiter
5. Iodine-induced hyperthyroidism
6. Iodism
7. Thyroid cancer

150

ALLERGY TO IODINE

In my experience, an allergy to inorganic iodine/iodide is a rare occurrence. An allergy to radioactive iodine dye, commonly used in many medical imaging procedures, does not guarantee an allergy to inorganic iodine/iodide (such as in Lugol's or Iodoral®). In fact, my experience has shown that it is a rare occurrence to have an allergy to inorganic iodine/iodide.

An allergy can take any form, including a rash, fatigue, congestion, headache, and fever. NAET, an acupressure technique, has been useful in some of my patients to help them overcome an allergy to iodine. More information on NAET can be found in Appendix A.

Joan, age 62, suffered from hypothyroidism for 20 years. Although Joan's symptoms improved on a holistic treatment plan (detoxification, vitamins and minerals, and diet change), she still was not feeling like she wanted to feel. When she was diagnosed with an iodine deficiency, I recommended that she take iodine. Joan was given an iodide/iodine supplement (Iodoral®) and immediately felt better. "It was like waking up from a nap. Within one week, my head felt clearer and my energy level improved. I have a busy job and I was having trouble keeping up with it," she said. Approximately two weeks after starting Iodoral®, Joan called me complaining of rash on her body. I told her to stop the iodine immediately. Joan told me, "I don't want to stop it. This is the first time in years that I have felt wonderful." I had Joan come into the office and treated her with NAET. Joan's allergy symptoms abated within 24 hours, and she is currently taking iodine without any problems. She continues to feel well today.

AUTOIMMUNE THYROID DISEASE

Some researchers and endocrinologists believe that autoimmune thyroid problems are caused by iodine intake in excess of the RDA. However, before the adoption of radioactive iodine to treat the side effects of autoimmune thyroid illnesses, the use of higher doses of iodine was the treatment of choice for these illnesses. There are numerous reports in the literature, some dating back well over 100 years, showing the benefits of using iodine in excess of the RDA to treat autoimmune thyroid illnesses.[2][3][4][5]

If iodine was the cause of autoimmune thyroid illnesses, these illnesses should have been decreasing over the last 30 years. The opposite has occurred. In the United States, iodine levels have fallen approximately 50% over the last 30 years while, at the same time, autoimmune thyroid disorders have been rapidly increasing.[6]

My clinical experience has shown that in an iodine deficient state, higher doses of iodine are an effective and safe way to treat autoimmune thyroid illness without appreciable side effects.

152

DETOXIFICATION REACTIONS

In Chapter 5, it was established that iodine could compete with the toxic halides, bromide and fluoride. The study I undertook showed that the use of iodine can result in the release of the toxic halides from the body (see Chapter 5). If the body's detoxification pathways are overloaded when the toxic halides are being released, a detoxification reaction can be triggered. A detoxification reaction can take the form of fatigue, muscle aches, fever, diarrhea, and brain fog, among others.

Though a detoxification reaction to iodine usage is rare, it has happened. A detoxification reaction can be minimized with using nutritional support (vitamins and minerals), balancing the hormonal system, getting the body's pH balanced, eating healthy foods, and other holistic treatments.

IODINE-INDUCED HYPOTHYROIDISM AND GOITER

When animals or humans that are iodine deficient are given large doses of iodine, there is a transient decrease in thyroid hormone production (approximately 26-40 hours) until the body reestablishes its equilibrium with iodine.[7][8] After that time, thyroid levels adjust to normal and signs of hypothyroidism do not develop.

Many researchers point out the dangers of iodine by describing the goiter problems of the residents of Hokkaido, Japan. A report in 1960 described how a significant portion of the population of Hokkaido, Japan had developed goiter. Goiters were more common in seaweed fishermen and in villages where seaweed was eaten in large quantities. The residents of Hokkaido, as well as other areas of Japan, were found to be ingesting large amounts of iodine. The Japanese authors did not think that iodine was the causative factor of the goiters since residents of inland areas had the same iodine intake as the residents in Hokkaido, and they had no signs of increased goiter. Clearly, some other factor must have been involved. Although no testing was done, goitrogens (such as bromide) could have caused the elevated goiter picture. A follow-up study 27 years later found a similar iodine intake in Hokkaido residents but no signs of excess goiter, therefore ruling out iodine as the cause.

I have spoken with other doctors who have used higher doses of iodine in the treatment of their patients; they also report no increase in hypothyroid or goiter problems.[9]

IODINE-INDUCED HYPERTHYROIDISM

The use of iodine in a previously iodine-deficient population may result in a transient increase in thyroid hormones. Studies have shown that the increase in thyroid hormones, which could lead to hyperthyroid symptoms (i.e., palpitations, nervousness), will gradually decrease.[10] These side effects can easily be monitored by routine lab tests and adjustments in dosages.

Researchers from Switzerland found that the correction of iodine deficiency not only decreased the incidence of thyrotoxicosis, it also lowered the incidence of goiter, cretinism, and minor deficiencies of intellect.[11] My experience has shown that iodine-induced hyperthyroidism is not a common occurrence.

IODISM

Iodism occurs when the dose of iodine is too high and results in a metallic taste in the mouth, increased salivation, sneezing, headache, and acne. Also, sinus headache, especially headache in the frontal area, and a sense of fever may be present. Iodism occurs in a small minority of patients and is easily rectified by adjusting the dosage of iodine used.

Dr. Sherry Tenpenny claims that chlorophyll tablets will eliminate the metallic taste of iodine. Dr. Flechas has reported similar results with chlorophyll.

THYROID CANCER

Thyroid cancers are a small minority of cancers in the United States representing 1% of all cancers.[12] Women are affected in larger numbers than men, approximately 3:1.

There have been some reports in the literature that iodine supplementation can be associated with an increased incidence of thyroid papillary cancer.[13] If iodine usage were the cause of

155

thyroid cancer, then the falling iodine levels would be expected to lead to lowered thyroid cancer levels. However, this has not been the case. During the past several decades, when iodine levels have declined, the incidence of thyroid cancer has markedly increased.[14] Perhaps iodine deficiency is the cause of the elevation in thyroid cancers.

Iodine supplementation has been shown to significantly improve the prognosis of thyroid cancer by shifting the type of cancer to a more easily treatable (i.e., differentiated) form.[15]

Radiation exposure has been positively correlated with thyroid cancer for over 50 years. Over the years, numerous studies have confirmed this link, including the problems at Chernobyl. One of the treatments for exposure to radiation is iodine. Potassium iodide was given to residents of Poland and Russia after the Chernobyl accident and has been hailed as a success in preventing more cases of thyroid cancer.

In an iodine deficient state, when exposed to radioactive iodine (such as in Chernobyl), the thyroid gland will absorb large amounts of the radioactive iodine. This will lead to thyroid cancer. However, if the thyroid gland is saturated with iodine, radioactive iodine will be absorbed at much smaller amounts and the problems with thyroid cancer will be lessened.

It makes perfect sense to have the body sufficient with iodine before being subjected to a toxic exposure of radioactive iodine.

HOW MUCH IODINE SHOULD YOU TAKE?

Now we are back to the question above. There is no perfect dose for everyone. The best way to properly dose iodine is to test the body for its iodine status. This can easily be accomplished with an iodine-loading test. The instructions for the loading test are detailed below.

Iodine-Loading Test
1. First morning urine is discarded.
2. Take 50mg of iodine/iodide (Iodoral®) with a glass of water.
3. Collect 24-hour urine. Include the first morning sample at the end of the 24-hour collection.
4. Send a sample of the 24-hour urine for evaluation of iodine status.

The principle behind using the iodine-loading test has been well established. If the body was saturated with iodine, one would expect that most of the 50mg of iodine ingested for the loading test would be excreted. If, on the other hand, there was an iodine deficiency present, then more of the iodine would be absorbed.

Research has shown that a 90% excretion (or 45mg of iodine) of a 50mg iodine-loading test would indicate an iodine sufficient state. Levels below 90% (or <45mg) would indicate an iodine deficiency state. In this case, iodine supplementation can begin and retesting can be performed in the future. To find out more about iodine testing, I refer the reader to FFP Labs: 877.900.5556.

Once an iodine-deficient state is determined, iodine supplementation can be implemented. I recommend using a combination of iodine and iodide. This can be found in liquid or tablet form. Appendix A will give you more information on how to find an iodine supplement.

Chapter 1 established that iodine concentrates in all of the trillions of cells in the body. Not only does it concentrate in the thyroid and breasts, it also accumulates in the prostate, salivary glands, skin, intestines, and all the red and white blood cells throughout the body. Proper iodine supplementation needs to address all of these issues. Approximately 12mg of iodine has been established as the optimal daily dose of iodine/iodide for the breast and thyroid gland. However, this may not be adequate to address the needs of the rest of the body.

Also, due to the contact with so many goitrogenic substances such as bromide and fluoride (see Chapter 5), the daily iodine requirements may be elevated for some. Depending on the iodine status of the body, my experience has shown that the RDA for iodine (150μg/day) is inadequate not only for the thyroid gland, but for the rest of the body as well. We live in a toxic society, and elevated amounts of goitrogens in our environment (in the form of bromine, fluoride, and chlorine derivatives) require a larger amount of iodine in order to achieve sufficiency. Although the dose should be individualized, my experience has shown that the dose can vary from 6-50mg/day for most adults. This is the daily dose that Dr. Guy Abraham recommends. I have often found an effective dose to be somewhere between 12 and 50mg per day. This higher iodine dose can easily be followed by an iodine-loading test and proper adjustments implemented depending on the clinical presentation.

SALIVA/SERUM IODIDE LEVELS

When iodine is taken orally, it is absorbed into the blood stream. Iodine is transported into the target cells of the body by an energy-dependant process. One atom of iodine is transported into the cells and two atoms of sodium are transported out of cells via the sodium/iodide symporter (NIS).[16] [17] Recently a second mechanism for transport of iodine into the cells has been observed—the chloride/iodide transporter known as pendrin.[18]

Iodine may be absorbed through the intestines resulting in an elevated serum level of iodine, but the target cells are unable to uptake the iodine. This can occur if the NIS and/or the pendrin transporter systems are damaged. Certain goitrogens, such as bromide, can bind to the NIS causing damage to the transport system. The end result of this damage would be iodine deficiency in the target cell. Dr. Abraham and I reported a case history of my nurse, Denise, who had a transport defect of iodine.[19]

Upon taking iodine orally, the iodine is absorbed in the intestine. As serum levels of iodine increase, iodine is transported into the target cells via the NIS or pendrin. One way to determine if the transport mechanism for iodine is working is by measuring the saliva/serum iodide ratio. If the transport mechanisms for iodine are properly functioning, the saliva levels of iodine will significantly increase relative to the serum. A saliva/serum iodide level has been used in neonates to diagnose a congenital iodide symporter defect.[20]

We (Dr. Abraham, Dr. Flechas and Dr. Brownstein) have been evaluating saliva/serum iodide levels in a series of patients. Initial results show that the normal saliva/serum iodide level is approximately 42. That means that when iodine is being properly transported into the cells, the salivary fluid should have 42 times the iodine level that is found in the serum. If the saliva/serum levels are low, especially less than 20, a thorough search for a reason for the poor transport of iodine must be undertaken.

Goitrogens can bind to and damage the NIS and result in a lowered amount of iodine being transported into the target cell.[21] Examples of these goitrogens include: fluoride, perchlorate, bromine, and thiocyanate (from cigarette smoke). In the near-future, saliva/serum iodine levels will be used to diagnose an iodine transport defect.

Bob, a 42-year-old accountant, had been taking 12.5mg of iodine/iodide for two years. Bob could not tell a difference upon taking the iodine. Although he felt generally well, he complained of being fatigued. His initial salivary/serum level was low at 9.3. Bob's testing also showed that his serum bromine levels were *elevated—147mg/L (normal <5mg/L). I increased Bob's iodine dosage to 50mg/day. Immediately, he felt a boost in his energy. "I thought I was feeling pretty good until I increased the iodine. Then I really felt good. After work I wasn't so exhausted," he said. Bob's follow-up testing showed that his salivary/serum iodide levels improved to a healthier 48.6 and his bromine level fell to 28.7mg/L.*

Bromine is a toxic halide that has no place in our bodies. Chapter 5 describes the problems with bromine in more detail. Bromine, being part of the halide family (along with iodine and fluoride) can not only compete and bind to the iodine receptors in the body, it can also damage the NIS and block the target cells' ability to absorb iodine. Due to our increasing exposure to the toxic halogens (i.e., bromine and fluoride), as well as our exposure to other goitrogens (perchlorate, thiocyanate, etc.), our need for iodine has actually increased. In Bob's case, a higher iodine intake was able to help his body overcome the bromine toxicity that was present.

We (Drs. Abraham and Brownstein) have reported on the repair of an iodine transport defect with the use of Vitamin C and unrefined sea salt (Celtic Sea Salt®).[22] This case study provides evidence that the damage to the iodine transport mechanism can be repaired with a complete nutritional program.

FINAL THOUGHTS

Iodine, like any substance, can cause adverse effects (mentioned above). For individuals who are unusually sensitive to supplements and medications, I would recommend starting with a low dose of iodine and titrating the dose upward. Close monitoring of the symptoms can often guide the dosage.

To lesson side effects, iodine supplementation is more effective when it is given as part of a complete nutritional program. My clinical experience has shown that balancing vitamins, minerals and hormones along with iodine supplementation provides a better result as compared to using iodine as a single agent.

[1] Nagataki, S. Thyroid function in chronic excess iodide ingestion: Comparison of thyroidal absolute iodine uptake and degradation of thyroxine in euthyroid Japanese subjects. J. Clin. Endo. 27:638-647, 1967

[2] Trousseau, A. Lectures on clinical medicine. Vol. 1. Lecture XIX, Exophthalmic goiter of Graves' disease, New Sydenham Society, London. 1868

[3] Thompson, W. Prolonged treatment of exophthalmic goiter by iodine alone. Arch. Int. Med. 45:481-502, 1930

[4] Plummer, H. Results of administering iodine to patients having exophthalmic goiter. JAMA. 1923;80: 1955

[5] Thompson, W. The range of effective iodine dosage in exophthalmic goiter. Arch. Int. Med. 1930;45:261-281

[6] Hollowell, JE et al. Iodine nutrition in the United States. Trends and public health implications: Iodine excretion data from National Health and Nutrition Examination Surveys I and III (1971-74 and 1988-94). J Clin Endocrinol Metab 83:3401-3408. 1998.

[7] Wolf, Jan. Iodide goiter and the pharmacologic effects of excess iodide. American Journal of Med. Vol. 47. July, 1969

[8] Wolff, J. The temporary nature of the inhibitory action of excess iodide on organic iodine synthesis in the normal thyroid. Endocrin. 45:504, 1949

[9] Personal communication with Dr. G. Abraham and Dr. J. Flechas

[10] Baltisberger, B. Decrease of incidence of toxic nodular goiter in a region of Switzerland after full correction of mild iodine deficiency. Eur. J. Endocrin. 1995;132:546

[11] Gurgi, G. Thyrotoxicosis incidence in Switzerland and benefit of improved iodine supply. Letter to the Editor. The Lancet. Vol. 352. September 26, 1998

[12] NIH pub. No. 96-4104. Bethesda, MD, 2000

[13] Harach, G. Thyroid cancer and thyroiditis in goitrous region of Salta, Argentina, before and after iodine prophylaxis. Clin. Endocrin. 1995;43: 701

[14] Schneider, Arthur. Carcinoma of follicular epithelium. In Werner and Ingbar's The Thyroid. Lippincott Wililams and Wilkins. 2000

[15] IBID. Schneider.

[16] Brown-Grant, K. Extrathyroidal iodide concentrating mechanism. Physiol. Rev. 41:1961

[17] Spitzweg, C. Analysis of human sodium iodide symporter immunoreactivity in human exocrine glands. J. Clin. Endocrin. And Metab. 84, 4178-4184 1999.

[18] Everett, L. Pendred syndrome is caused by a mutation in a putative sulphate transporter gene. Nat. Genet. 17:1997

[19] Abraham,G and Brownstein, D. Evidence that the administration of Vitamin C improves a defective cellular transport mechanism for iodine: A case report. TheOriginal Internist. Vol. 12, No. 3. Fall 2005. 125-130.

[20] Viljder, J. Hereditary metabolic disorders causing hypothyroidism. In Werner and Ingbar's the Thyroid. Braverman, LE et al. Lippincott Williams and Wilkins, 733-742, 2000.

[21] Abraham, G.E. The historical background of the iodine project. The Original Internist. 12(2):57-66 2005 57-66

[22] Abraham, G., Brownstein, D. Evidence that the administration of Vitamin C improves a defective cellular transport mechanism for iodine: A Case Report. The Original Internist. 2005;12(3):125-130

Chapter 8

Questions and Answers

CHAPTER EIGHT: QUESTIONS AND ANSWERS

This chapter will help to answer common questions regarding iodine.

Q: *Is iodine deficiency more prevalent now than it was in the past?*

A: *Although we have lived in an iodine-poor environment, iodine deficiency is probably more pronounced now due to the increased toxicity of our modern surroundings. The onslaught of chemicals and goitrogens such as bromine and fluoride has risen dramatically over the last 30 years. Goitrogens can bind to iodine receptors and also bind to and damage the transport mechanisms for iodine. Goitrogens can exacerbate the iodine deficiency problem that already is present. Combined with a declining nutrient level in our food, it is no wonder that people require higher iodine levels than in the past.*

Q: *Does iodine cause autoimmune thyroid illness such as Hashimoto's and Graves' disease?*

A: No. Autoimmune thyroid illnesses have been increasing over the last 30 years, while iodine levels have been falling. If iodine was the cause of autoimmune thyroid illness, as iodine levels fall, you would expect to see a decline in the incidence of Hashimoto's and Graves' disease, which has not happened.

Q: Are there side effects with iodine supplementation?

A: There are potential side effects from supplementing with anything, iodine included. With proper follow-up visits and monitoring, adverse effects are easily treated. Chapter 7 reviews the adverse effects of iodine in more detail.

Q: Why hasn't conventional medicine recognized that iodine deficiency is still present today?

A: A natural product cannot be patented. A patentable product can be very profitable for a pharmaceutical company. Their main interest is to make a profit. Big Pharma has shown little interest in any natural product because they cannot maximize their profits on non-patentable products. Furthermore, most of the money for drug research is controlled by pharmaceutical companies. Big Pharma has no financial interest in looking at any natural product, including iodine.

Q: Does iodine supplementation cause goiter?

A: No. Iodine deficiency causes goiter, not iodine supplementation. Medical research has shown this for over 100 years.

Q: Does iodine deficiency cause breast cancer?

A: Breast cancer is a multi-factorial illness. However, the evidence linking iodine deficiency to breast cancer is overwhelming. Iodine deficiency may not be the sole cause of the epidemic of breast cancer that is plaguing us today, but, it plays a very large role in this illness. I do not think you can adequately treat a chronic illness like breast cancer without looking for the underlying cause(s). Breast cancer is not caused by a deficiency of chemotherapy, radiation and surgery. I have no doubt that iodine deficiency, coupled with the increased toxic load of our environment, is a major part of the reason why we have an epidemic of breast cancer.

Q: Don't I get enough iodine from salt?

A: No. The iodine in salt is not very bioavailable for our bodies. In addition, many people are avoiding salt entirely in their diets. Refined salt is a toxic substance for our bodies and needs to be avoided. For more information, I refer the reader to my book, Salt Your Way to Health.

Q: Can I get too much iodine?

A: Yes. You can get too much of anything. It is essential to have proper follow-up with your health care provider. As previously stated, excess iodine levels can easily be treated with an adjustment of the dose.

Q: Do I have to lower the dose of my thyroid medication when I start taking iodine?

A: It varies for everybody, but, my experience has shown that one-third of the people being treated with thyroid hormone can lower or significantly reduce their level of thyroid hormone when starting iodine. The other two-thirds of the people taking thyroid hormone can remain on the same dosage. If there are any palpitations when starting iodine, decrease the thyroid dose immediately.

Q: Does iodine supplementation cause palpitations?

A: In some people it does. Iodine supplementation works best as part of a holistic treatment regimen emphasizing vitamins, minerals, and hormone balancing. Some patients are very sensitive to everything they take. Sometimes I have my patients take iodine every other day. Each person needs an individualized dose.

Q: Is iodine an antioxidant?

A: The research is clear; iodine can function as both an antioxidant and an oxidant. We need a balance in our bodies between both antioxidants and oxidants. Iodine, like Vitamin C, can help to provide this balance. This topic was covered in more detail in Chapter 5.

Chapter 9

Case Histories

CHAPTER 9: CASE HISTORIES

This chapter will contain several case histories that will illustrate how iodine deficiency is recognized and treated. It will also provide the practitioner with information on how to approach the patient with iodine deficiency.

Betty is an 82-year-old female who has a twenty-five year history of thyroid nodules and intermittent hyperthyroid symptoms. Betty was advised to receive radioactive iodine to treat her condition, but she refused. As explained in Chapter 6, radioactive iodine does not treat any underlying cause of a thyroid illness. I believe that radioactive iodine should be the last choice in treating any thyroid disorder.

Betty was given an iodine loading test with 50mg of iodine/iodide (Iodoral®). Her initial iodine loading test showed a

very low iodine excretion with a 35% excretion measured (normal
>90%). Betty's initial thyroid ultrasound showed an enlarged
thyroid gland with a total volume of 13.1ml. She also had large
nodules in both the right and left lobes of the thyroid gland.

Betty was placed on 50mg/day of iodine/iodide (Iodoral®).
Betty was also placed on Vitamin C, unrefined sea salt (Celtic Sea
Salt®) and magnesium. The Vitamin C can function as an
antioxidant and can help support the body's detoxification
pathways. Celtic Sea Salt® can supply the body with chloride
which aids in detoxifying toxic halides (bromide and fluoride).
Celtic Sea Salt® is also a good source of minerals. Magnesium is
a relaxing agent for the body and can help prevent hyperthyroid
symptoms caused by a detoxification of toxic halides.

After two months of taking 50mg/day of iodine/iodide
(Iodoral®), Betty felt much better. Her energy improved and she
felt that her brain fog had resolved. A repeat thyroid ultrasound
showed the size of the thyroid gland decreased to 10.3ml—a 22%
decline. In addition, all of the nodules were noted to be smaller
from the previous ultrasound. Betty's thyroid levels were
unchanged from taking 50mg of iodine.

Before the usage of iodine/iodide in milligram doses, it was
rare to see thyroid nodules and a hypertrophied thyroid gland
shrink in size. Now it is common in my practice. Only with the
proper dose of iodine/iodide (in mg doses) have I found thyroid
nodules to recede.

David is a 48-year-old health club owner. David was diagnosed with thyroid cancer ten years ago and had a thyroidectomy followed by chemotherapy. He was placed on Synthroid and had his dose of Synthroid titrated until his thyroid levels showed a euthyroid state. However, after the surgery, David gained 50 pounds of weight and never felt the same. "I exercised all the time and I couldn't lose an ounce. It did not matter whether I ate or not. I kept telling my doctors that I did not feel right—I was always tired and I couldn't think straight," he said. When I saw David, his physical exam showed a slight edematous feeling around the lower neck in the area of his thyroidectomy. David claimed, "I always told my doctor that I felt something around my neck. They kept telling me that nothing was there since I had my thyroid removed." An iodine loading test showed David was extremely low in iodine—he had one of the lowest loading tests that I have seen-- 0.3% excretion (normal >90%). David was also found to be excreting large amounts of the toxic halide bromide (see figure on next page). Bromide is a toxic element and no bromide should be present in the body. David was started on 50mg of iodine/iodide (Iodoral®), and his iodine and bromide levels were reevaluated at 1 day and 30 days. His results are seen in the figure on the next page. Due to the large amounts of bromide, David was treated with a holistic regimen designed to support his detoxification pathways. This included Vitamin C, unrefined salt (Celtic Sea Salt®), and liver support. Two months later he reported, "My brain fog cleared and I began to lose *weight for the first time since the surgery. It is a miracle." Also, the edema around the lower neck resolved and David no longer felt as if his neck was being squeezed.*

Case History David: Iodide/Bromide Levels Before and After Iodine Supplementation

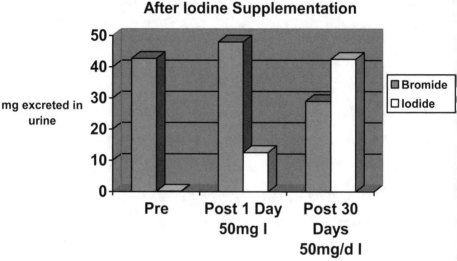

Iodine deficiency is associated with hypertrophy of the thyroid gland as well as hyperplasia of the thyroid gland. Often times, when there is iodine deficiency present, the physical exam will reveal an edematous feeling in the thyroid area of the neck, often like there are "cotton balls" surrounding the thyroid gland. Patients will often report to me that they have a swollen feeling of the thyroid gland. Most times, when the iodine deficiency is rectified, the edematous feeling will resolve. The treatment for thyroid cancer must include identifying and treating the underlying cause(s) of the illness. The conventional approach to thyroid cancer relies on the use of surgery, chemotherapy and radiation. However, thyroid cancer does not develop because of a deficiency of thyroid surgery, radiation or chemotherapy. A treatment can only be effective if it treats the underlying cause(s) of the condition. Research has shown that iodine can induce apoptosis (programmed cell death) of thyroid cancer cells.[1]

As stated previously, there is no doubt that iodine deficiency plays a large role in the development of thyroid cancer (as well as other cancers). Only with rectifying iodine deficiency, coupled with a comprehensive treatment plan that emphasizes optimizing the function of the immune system, will people be able to prevent and overcome these serious disorders.

Janice, a 52-year-old nurse (my nurse) was complaining of intermittent fatigue and muscle aches. At the beginning of our work day, I could tell how Janice was feeling by the way she walked down the hall. If she was feeling well, she had a bounce in her step. If she was feeling down, she would have a slight slouch to her body and slowness in her step. Usually by the end of a busy day, Janice would be extremely fatigued and complain of muscle and joint pain. "Sometimes my feet and legs would just be killing me by the end of the day," she said. Janice was very sensitive to all medications and supplements. She frequently took children's doses of items because she had such a sensitive system. She did not want to do an iodine loading test because she feared taking the loading dose of iodine—50mg. I elected to therapeutically treat her with 12.5mg of iodine/iodide (Iodoral®). Immediately, she felt better. "All of my pain was gone in three days. After two weeks, my energy zoomed higher. I was no longer aching at the end of the work day; I felt great," she claimed. After four weeks of taking 12.5mg Iodoral®/day, she developed mild palpitations. I told her to stop the iodine and the palpitations subsided one day later. Janice was instructed to take 12.5mg Iodoral® three days per week. In addition, she was placed on a vitamin and mineral regimen. Janice did well for the next five months until one day at work I saw her limping down the hall. I asked her why she was limping and she told me, "I feel terrible. Everything aches and my feet are killing me." When I asked her if she was taking the iodine, she told me that she quit it one week ago. Incredulously, I asked her "why?" She told me that she thought she had enough in her body. After a few terse comments, I instructed her to resume the iodine dose. By the time Janice had taken her third iodine dose, all of her symptoms again resolved.

Shirley, at 69-years-old is very sensitive to medications and supplements. She also happens to be my mother-in-law. Shirley was on 6.25mg/day of iodine/iodide (Iodoral®) to help treat many hypothyroid symptoms including cold extremities, hair loss, dry skin, and fatigue. All of her symptoms improved significantly with the iodine supplementation. Furthermore, she was able to stop taking thyroid hormone due to the positive effects of the iodine. Approximately four months after starting the iodine regimen,

178

Shirley developed palpitations. Now, having your mother-in-law develop palpitations is not a good thing. The palpitations ceased after two days without the iodine. Shirley was instructed to take microgram doses of iodine in the form of Atomidine® (Edgar Cayce's iodine formulation) three days per week. Since reducing her dose, all of her hypothyroid symptoms have improved and she is not having palpitations. Shirley's case is very rare. I have only had to use microgram amounts of iodine three times over the last 3.5 years. This has only occurred in patients extremely sensitive to nearly everything.

The above cases illustrate that every patient needs to have an individualized treatment plan. Those that are sensitive to medications may need a lowered dose, and may need to titrate their dose of iodine. If one is deficient in iodine, it is rare not to be able to find an appropriate dose to improve the clinical condition.

Amanda, a 23-year-old fitness instructor, complained of coldness of her extremities and fatigue. "I teach four aerobic classes per day and I am exhausted after each class," she said. Amanda's saliva/serum of iodide could not be calculated since her iodine level was too low. In addition, she was found to have a large amount of bromide in her serum (127mg/L). As established in Chapter 5, bromide is a toxic halogen that inhibits iodine absorption and binding in the body. Amanda was started on 25mg/day of iodine/iodide (Iodoral®). Immediately, her symptoms improved. "I was not exhausted after teaching my aerobics class.

179

Also, my hands and feet warmed up," she said. Amanda was also complaining of a rash on her skin after teaching a pool aerobics class. The pool was sanitized with bromine. After taking the iodine, the rash immediately disappeared. Follow-up testing revealed that Amanda's saliva/serum iodide improved to 42.5 and her serum bromine level fell to 16.7mg/L.

Amanda's case is very common. The correction of iodine deficiency can resolve the symptoms of hypothyroidism. In fact, if there is iodine deficiency and hypothyroidism present, iodine deficiency needs to be corrected first. This was explained in Chapter 6. In Amanda's case, correcting an iodine deficit was probably helping the body rid itself of the toxic halide bromine. The improvement in her skin was evidence of this.

Kim, a 42 year old business woman wanted desperately to have another child. She said, "My son is 11 and I want him to have a brother or sister." Kim had two miscarriages over the last two years and she had a difficult time getting pregnant. Her first pregnancy was very hard for her as she was extremely fatigued and had a very difficult delivery. Kim was diagnosed with hypothyroidism after the birth of her first child and placed on thyroid hormone (Armour thyroid). "I did feel better with the Armour thyroid, but I was still cold. The worst thing was that my energy never really returned after the birth of my son," she said. Kim heard a lecture that I gave on iodine and had her iodine levels checked. Her iodine-loading test was low at 22% excretion (normal >90%) and she was placed on 50mg/day of Iodoral®. "I felt a huge change immediately. My energy returned and all of my remaining hypothyroid symptoms resolved within weeks. It felt like a miracle," she said. Kim became pregnant shortly after starting the iodine supplementation and she delivered a healthy baby boy 9 months later. During the pregnancy, she continued the iodine supplement. "At 42 years old, this was the easiest pregnancy. I gained 16 pounds and could fit into all my regular clothes right after I delivered. My midwife was amazed at how easy this pregnancy was on me. I wasn't even fatigued after the delivery. I wish that I had taken iodine earlier in my life," she claimed.

Kim's story is not unique. Iodine supplementation can help the improve a hypothyroid condition. Many times, even with the supplementation of thyroid hormone, hypothyroid some hypothyroid symptoms still remain. My experience has shown that the best results in treating a thyroid condition will occur when iodine deficiency is rectified.

[1] Vitale, M. Endocrinology. 141.

Chapter 10

Final Thoughts

CHAPTER 10: FINAL THOUGHTS

This book was written to educate the reader on the benefits and the importance of iodine. In medical school, the only mention of iodine that I recall was that iodized salt corrected iodine deficiency, and that radioactive iodine was useful for treating thyroid cancer. Iodine deficiency was only mentioned as a thing of the past.

I have found iodine deficiency occurring in a surprisingly large number of my patients. When I started checking my patients for their iodine status, I expected to find a large percentage of patients deficient. However, I was stunned to find over 90% of my patients have consistently tested deficient in iodine.

In my practice, I have found that iodine supplementation (when indicated) has helped numerous conditions including fatigue states, autoimmune disorders, and cancer. In addition, iodine supplementation significantly improves hormonal imbalances including hypothyroidism and Hashimoto's and Graves' disease. Iodine supplementation works best when used in conjunction with a comprehensive holistic treatment plan, including the use of natural items such as vitamins, minerals and hormones.

Chapter 1 describes the history of iodine and how the link between goiter and iodine deficiency was established. The addition of iodine to salt was a major medical success in significantly improving cretinism and reducing the prevalence of goiter. However, iodized salt has not been enough to correct iodine deficiency.

Chapter 2 reviews why iodized salt is insufficient in maintaining adequate iodine levels. One of the biggest mistakes in the history of modern food processing (amongst many mistakes) has been the substitution of bromine for iodine in the manufacturing of bread and pastry products. This has certainly contributed to the declining level of our health as a society. It is no wonder that iodine-deficient disorders such as breast cancer, prostate cancer, and autoimmune disorders are rising at epidemic rates.

Iodine supplementation must be given with the correct form of iodine. Chapter 3 reviews why an iodine supplement should contain both iodine and iodide.

Breast cancer and fibrocystic breast illness are covered in Chapter 4. The medical literature is replete with information relating the rise in breast cancer to iodine deficiency. Though I think breast cancer can be a multifactorial problem, I have no doubt that iodine deficiency is a significant piece of the puzzle in the breast cancer epidemic that is presently occurring.

The connection between declining iodine levels and the toxic halides, bromine, fluoride, and perchlorate are covered in more detail in Chapter 5. There is compelling evidence that the toxic halides should be avoided at all costs.

Thyroid disorders are closely tied to the iodine status in the individual. Chapter 6 describes the range of thyroid problems that develop with inadequate iodine levels. This includes hypothyroidism and Hashimoto's and Graves' disease. The fear of supplementing with iodine in thyroid disorders is unfounded when there is proper medical supervision.

Chapter 7 gives the reader information on how much iodine to take. This chapter was written to reassure the reader that the proper use and monitoring of iodine is safe. The fallacy of using radioactive iodine as the first line of treatment for hyperthyroid and autoimmune thyroid problems is also covered. Ensuring adequate iodine supplementation should be the first line of treatment for these disorders.

Common question and answers are covered in Chapter 8. The questions presented are the most common questions I hear from health care providers and patients alike.

Case histories are reviewed in Chapter 9. This chapter will provide the reader with actual case histories and why it is so important to check iodine levels.

Chapter 10 discusses several case histories and how these patients responded to iodine. These are some examples of the effectiveness of orthoiodosupplementation.

Iodine is one of the most important minerals in the body. It is crucial to have your iodine levels checked and supplemented with the correct form of iodine, when indicated. Taking iodine can mean the difference between optimal health and illness.

To All of Our Health!!!

APPENDIX A: RESOURCES

1. Iodoral® can be purchased from:

> Optimox Research Corporation
> 2720 Monterey Street
> Ste. 406
> Torrance, CA 90503
> 1.800.223.1601

2. For iodine testing and the iodine-loading test as well as bromide and fluoride testing contact:

> FFP Lab
> 500 S. Allen Rd.
> Ste. #1
> Flat Rock, NC 28731
> 1.877.900.5556

2. For allergies to iodine, NAET (Nambudripod's Allergy Elimination Technique) can be helpful. To find an NAET practitioner   please call: 1.714.523.3068 or look on the internet: www.naet.com.

3. A compounding pharmacist can make up Lugol's solution. To find a compounding pharmacist please contact:

> The International Academy of Compounding Pharmacists (IACP)
> P.O. Box 1365
> Sugar Land, TX 77487
> iacpinfo@iacprx.org
> (800)-927-4227
> Fax: 281-495-0602

Glossary

Adrenal glands: Either of a pair of endocrine organs located on top of the kidneys, which produce hormones, including DHEA and hydrocortisone.

Antioxidant: A substance that opposes oxidation reactions. These substances are believed to help reduce damage in the body caused by free radicals.

Bromide: Any binary compound of bromine in which the bromine carries a negative electrical charge (Br^-). Bromides produce depression of the central nervous system, and were once widely used for their sedative effect.

Bromine: A reddish-brown liquid element. Gives off suffocating vapors. Its atomic number is 35.

Bromism: A condition of poisoning produced by the excessive use of bromine or bromine compound. It is characterized by neurological symptoms such as mental dullness, deficiency memory, slurred speech, drowsiness, unsteady gait, and by skin eruptions of various forms and fetor of breath.

Chloride: A binary compound of chlorine. The reduced form of chlorine, with an extra electron.

Chlorine: A yellowish green, gaseous element of suffocating odor. It is a disinfectant, decolorant, and an irritant poison. It is used for disinfecting, fumigating, and bleaching.

Detoxification: The process of removing toxins from the body.

Endocrine gland: A gland that produces an endocrine secretion commonly referred to as a hormone.

Estrogen: An entire group or class of steroid hormones produced primarily in the ovary; small amounts are also produced in the adrenal glands, testes and placenta. The three major forms of estrogen active in the female body are estrone, estradiol and estriol. Estrogen promotes the development of female secondary sex characteristics.

Fluoride: A binary compound of fluorine. Topically applied to the teeth as a dental caries' prophylactic.

Fluorine: A nonmetallic, gaseous element, belonging to the halogen family. Fluorine, in the form of fluoride is incorporated into the structure of bone and teeth. An excess of fluorine can result in fluorosis.

Halogen: An element of a closely related chemical family, all of which form similar (saltlike) compounds in combination with sodium and most other metals. The halogens are bromine, chlorine, fluorine, iodine and astatine.

Hormone: A product of living cells that circulates in the body fluids and produces a specific effect on the activity of cells remote from its point of origin.

Hyperthyroidism: Excessive production of thyroid hormone, resulting in an increased metabolic rate, tachycardia and high blood pressure.

Hypothalamus: A part of the brain that sits above the pituitary gland. It serves as the link between the nervous system and the hormonal or endocrine system.

Hypothyroidism: Inadequate production or utilization of thyroid hormone resulting in a myriad of symptoms including fatigue, a sense of coldness, atherosclerosis, menstrual irregularities, dry skin and others.

Inorganic: In chemistry, denoting substances not derived from hydrocarbons.

Menopause: The cessation of menstruation. Usually occurs between the ages of 46 and 55.

Organic: Denoting chemical substances containing carbon.

Osteoporosis: A condition characterized by a decrease in bone mass, resulting in porous and fragile bones. Hormonal imbalances and nutrient deficiencies are thought to lead to this condition.

Perchlorate: Consists of one atom of chlorine surrounded by four atoms of oxygen. It is a natural or man-made chemical. One of the main uses of perchlorate is as an explosive propellant for rockets. Perchlorate is a contaminate in water.

Pharmacologic doses: Refers to using doses of medications that exceed the body's own production of the particular substance. These high doses may make the body shut off its own production of the substance, resulting in the body becoming dependant on the exogenous source of that substance. Pharmacologic doses will lead to an increased chance of adverse side effects.

Physiologic doses: Refers to doses of medications that do not exceed the body's own intrinsic production of the substance. Physiologic doses do not shut off the body's own production of the substance. The chances of negative side effects are much reduced when using physiologic versus pharmacologic doses.

Pituitary: A small vascular endocrine organ located in the brain that regulates hormones which directly or indirectly affect most bodily functions.

Progesterone: A hormone produced by the adrenal glands and the ovaries. It is integral to the menstrual cycle and pregnancy. Progesterone imbalances are often associated with premenstrual syndrome and osteoporosis.

Premenstrual syndrome (PMS): A syndrome often associated with too little of the hormone progesterone and a resulting imbalance between estrogen and progesterone. Symptoms include cramps, depression, emotional swings, painful breasts, food cravings, weight gain and bloating.

Steroids: Any of numerous compounds containing a 17-carbon 4-ring system, including a variety of hormones. They have a common structure based on the steroid nucleus.

Testosterone: One of several anabolic, steroidal hormones produced by the adrenal cortex. When males reach puberty, the testes take over testosterone production and significantly increase its output. It has androgenic or masculinizing effects.

Index

X

Xenoestrogens 78

Other Books by Dr. Brownstein

The Guide to Healthy Eating
- What Food Should You Buy?
- What Food Should You Eat?
- What Food Should You Avoid?

Food is our best medicine. This book answers your questions about making healthy food choices and shopping for healthy, nutritional food. This book will serve as a helpful tool to guide you toward a wholesome meal ideas for you and your family.

The Miracle of Natural Hormones 3rd Edition
- Natural Progesterone
- DHEA
- Natural Testosterone
- Pregnenolone
- Other Natural Hormones

Dr. Brownstein describes his success with using safe and effective natural bioidentical hormones to treat illness and improve health.

Overcoming Thyroid Disorders
- Graves'
- Hashimoto's
- Hypothyroidism

This is a ground-breaking book on how to holistically treat thyroid disorders. See how a NATURAL approach to treating thyroid disorders is safe and effective.

Overcoming Arthritis

- **Holistic Treatment Program To Overcome Chronic Illness**
- **Rheumatoid Arthritis**
- **Fibromyalgia**
- **Chronic Fatigue Syndrome**
- **Over 30 Case Studies**
- **And Much More!!!**

Salt Your Way To Health

The myths of salt are dispelled in this book. This book will show you why salt is the most misunderstood nutrient. Unrefined salt is an integral part of a healthy diet. Refined salt is a toxic product that needs to be avoided. Read this book and learn about how salt can improve your health! See how adding the right kind of salt can help:

- **Adrenal Disorders**
- **Blood Pressure**
- **Cholesterol Levels**
- **Fatigue**
- **Headaches**
- **Immune System Function**
- **Thyroid Disorders**

Call 1-888-647-5616 or send a check or money order for:

Iodine: Why You Need It, Why You Can't Live Without It	$15.00
Miracle of Natural Hormones 3rd Edition	$15.00
Overcoming Arthritis	$15.00
Overcoming Thyroid Disorders	$15.00
Salt Your Way To Health	$15.00
The Guide To Healthy Eating	$15.00

Sales Tax: For Michigan residents, please add $.90 per book.

Shipping: 1 -2 Books: $4.00

3 Books: $3.00

4 Books: $2.00

5 Books: FREE SHIPPING!

VOLUME DISCOUNTS AVAILABLE. CALL 1-888-647-5616 FOR MORE INFORMATION OR ORDER ON-LINE AT: WWW.DRBROWNSTEIN.COM

Also, a NEW 2-Hour video by Dr. Brownstein is available describing his success in using natural therapies. The video is also available in DVD. The price is $30 (includes S+H).

Check or money orders can be sent to:
Medical Alternatives Press
4173 Fieldbrook
West Bloomfield, MI 48323